On Neurogenic Communication Disorders:

Original Short Stories and Case Studies

Second Edition

Dennis C. Tanner, Ph.D.

Professor of Health Sciences

Northern Arizona University

AUTHORS CHOICE PRESS

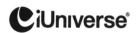

ON NEUROGENIC COMMUNICATION DISORDERS:
ORIGINAL SHORT STORIES AND CASE STUDIES
SECOND EDITION

Copyright © 2010, 2012, 2014 Dennis C. Tanner, Ph.D.

All rights reserved. No part of this book may be used or reproduced by any means graphic, electronic, or mechanical, including photocopying, recording, taping or by any information storage retrieval system without the written permission of the publisher except in the case of brief quotations embodied in critical articles and reviews.

The case studies provided herein are based on real persons and actual events. For confidentiality purposes, identifying information has been changed. Literary license has also been taken for descriptive and readability purposes. The people and institutions in the short stories are fictional and resemblance to real people and institutions is purely coincidental and unintentional.

AUTHORS CHOICE PRESS

iUniverse books may be ordered through booksellers or by contacting:

iUniverse LLC
1663 Liberty Drive
Bloomington, IN 47403
www.iuniverse.com
1-800-Authors (1-800-288-4677)

Originally published by Kendall Hunt Publishing Company

Because of the dynamic nature of the Internet, any web addresses or links contained in this book may have changed since publication and may no longer be valid. The views expressed in this work are solely those of the author and do not necessarily reflect the views of the publisher, and the publisher hereby disclaims any responsibility for them.

Any people depicted in stock imagery provided by Thinkstock are models, and such images are being used for illustrative purposes only. Certain stock imagery © Thinkstock.

ISBN: 978-1-4759-4867-7 (sc)
ISBN: 978-1-4759-6948-1 (e)

Printed in the United States of America.

iUniverse rev. date: 09/18/2014

Cover image © Artville

This book is dedicated to the memory of my father,
Ivan L. Tanner, a farmer, rancher, pilot, and gentleman.

Contents

Foreword

On Neurogenic Communication Disorders: Original Short Stories and Case Studies addresses neurogenic communication disorders in a unique and interesting way. It covers neurogenic communication disorders accurately while avoiding technical and clinical terminology where possible.

"Reflections on Global Aphasia" captures the struggle many patients undergo in coping and dealing with this communication disorder. "A Trip to the Fire Station," "The Reunion," "Cautious Clyde's Descent into Darkness," and "Traumatic Brain Injury" deal with the major cognitive, emotional, and communication disorders seen in many patients with serious head injuries. "Murphy's Inner World of Aphasia: Beth's Story" includes a spouse's perspective on aphasia and complements "Murphy's Inner World of Aphasia." "Alternately Abled" depicts several neurological disorders accurately and positively, with an interesting story line and plot. Other short stories and case studies concern stroke-related swallowing disorders and alternative treatment practices.

All in all, I found *On Neurogenic Communication Disorders: Original Short Stories and Case Studies* to be a unique and refreshing look into these serious disorders. It should provide readers, be they students, family members, or friends of patients, with insights and unique perspectives on these communication disorders that cannot be found in traditional academic and clinical texts.

Stephen Ritland, M.D.
Neurosurgeon

Preface

On Neurogenic Communication Disorders: Original Short Stories and Case Studies is a unique book. It is a collection of short stories and case studies about persons with neurogenic communication disorders. The short stories are based on people I have known as friends, acquaintances, or patients. The characters in the short stories are based on one person or a composite of several individuals. I have placed these characters in interesting fictional situations which provide a vehicle for showing their mettle in dealing with communication disorders and life challenges. The case studies are based on actual clinical cases and situations, but literary license has been taken to make them reader-friendly and interesting.

This book of short stories and case studies is not a scholarly clinical treatise on neurogenic communication disorders nor does it aspire to be one. While I believe it provides accurate information about neurogenic communication disorders, it is a work of fiction and simply a vehicle for understanding these complex and often devastating medical conditions.

Having taught at the university level for more than three decades, I have found students relate to this type of information presentation. Many find it a refreshing break from the sterile, clinical textbooks on neurogenic communication disorders they are required to read. I also believe that friends and family of persons afflicted with these disorders will gain insight from reading the book. Certainly, not every short story and case study will be relevant to all readers, but perhaps one or more of them will be worth the read.

To the Reader

On Neurogenic Communication Disorders: Original Short Stories and Case Studies is intended to be a brief, inexpensive supplement for courses in aphasia, motor speech disorders, and traumatic brain injury. I also believe these short stories and case studies will be of interest to friends and family of persons suffering from neurogenic communication disorders.

"The Silent Tongue (aphasia)" was authored by an award-winning poet after her sister suffered a stroke. It captures the despair and hope this nurse felt about her sister and aphasia.

"Reflections on Global Aphasia" deals with the devastation of the complete loss of language: global aphasia. I have seen hundreds of patients who have suffered this major, life-changing event. I have often wondered how persons deprived of language "think" and cope with the disorder. This case study draws from my interactions with these individuals, and chronicles what I believe to be the journey toward acceptance of life as a global aphasic person.

"A Trip to the Fire Station" is based on an actual misdiagnosis of post-traumatic psychosis. This case study involves a traumatic brain-injured patient in a nursing home, as well as several other patients being seen in group therapy. It illustrates the importance of understanding aphasic paraphasias in the proper diagnosis of traumatic brain injury.

"The Reunion" is a fact-based account of the devastation of a traumatic brain injury to a young couple on their honeymoon. It describes the major cognitive, behavioral, and emotional changes occurring in the groom following a tragic automobile accident, and the retrograde amnesia that eventually destroyed the newlywed's marriage.

"Cautious Clyde's Descent into Darkness" is an account of the effects of a traumatic brain injury resulting from an airplane accident. The traumatic brain injury sustained by the pilot is detailed, including problems with executive mental control.

"Crossed Aphasia in a Dextral: The Brain Localization Debate" is a discussion of an unusual type of aphasia resulting from damage to the right hemisphere of the brain. Included in this case study is a debate about the hotly contested brain localization movement.

"Traumatic Brain Injury" is a short story about post-traumatic psychosis, disorientation, and paranoid delusions. While it is impossible to truly know the thought processes of a patient so afflicted, this story attempts to depict severe traumatic brain injury from several perspectives.

"A Case of Severe Anterograde Amnesia" is a short vignette of a patient with severe impairments to storing new memories. Although anterograde amnesia is frequently caused by traumatic brain injury, her forgetfulness was the result of a stroke. The woman's amnesia was so severe that there was virtually no retention of new information for longer than a few minutes.

"Past Tense" uses time-travel as a vehicle to describe the arduous, if not brutal, treatment of persons with disabilities in the not-so-distant past. In this short story, a person with cerebral palsy and dysarthria is transported back in time to London, England in the late 1800s.

"The Peyote Way" is a description of a Native American alternative treatment for aphasia. It is a culturally sensitive exploration of one of the healing rites of the Native American Church performed on an aphasic person. (Permissions were obtained for a nonmember observer and there was a tribal government representative present to ensure appropriate witnessing and reporting of the ceremony.)

"Murder Challenged" is the fictional story of a professor with cerebral palsy and an attempt on his life. While addressing his dysarthric speech, this short story also delves into his experiences, thoughts, and emotions about dating, marriage, and interpersonal relationships.

I wrote "Murphy's Inner World of Aphasia" in the mid-1990s. It was originally published in my self-help book: *The Family Guide to Surviving Stroke and Communication Disorders* (Pearson Allyn & Bacon Publishers). This short story chronicles a stroke survivor's experiences with aphasia from the first onset of symptoms to discharge from a rehabilitation unit. Based on reader suggestions, I published "Murphy's Inner World of Aphasia: Beth's Story," in the second edition of *The Family Guide to Surviving Stroke and Communication Disorders* (Jones and Bartlett Publishers) to offer the perspective of Murphy's wife on this life-altering event. Together, these two short stories give the reader likely perspectives of stroke and aphasia from both the aphasic person and his wife.

"Alternately Abled" is a short story about the residents of a group home on an Alaskan adventure. Several of the characters in the story have neurogenic communication disorders. This story portrays them and their disabilities in a crisis situation.

"Preponderance of Evidence" gives introductory students an idea of what the practice of speech-language pathology is like in a medical environment. Several neurogenic communication disorders are depicted in this short story.

"A Day at JFK" chronicles a typical school day for teachers and students at an elementary school. It focuses on the activities of the speech-language pathologist.

"Welcome to the Cyber Speech and Hearing Clinic" provides insight into what the profession of speech-language pathology and audiology might look like in the not-so-distant future.

The short stories in this book are designed to portray persons with neurogenic communication disorders accurately and positively. I have attempted to do this while providing an interesting plot and story line from which I could develop their characters. The case studies are based on clinical events I observed during my career as a professor, scientist, and clinician. My goal in writing this book is to provide students, family members, and friends of persons with neurogenic communication disorders with a novel and refreshing vehicle for understanding these oftentimes devastating disabilities.

Dennis C. Tanner
June 8, 2014

About the Author

Dennis C. Tanner received the Doctor of Philosophy degree in Audiology and Speech Sciences from Michigan State University. Professor Tanner has 14 books in print, many of them addressing neurogenic communication disorders. He has published several journal articles and presented papers on neurogenic communication disorders and is coauthor of the Quick Assessment Series for Neurogenic Communication Disorders. Dr. Tanner has been named Outstanding Educator by the Association of Schools of Allied Health Professions and has been the College of Health Profession's Teacher of the Year. He serves as an expert witness in legal cases involving communication sciences and disorders, and is currently a Professor of Health Sciences at Northern Arizona University in Flagstaff, Arizona. For more information, visit his website: www.drdennistanner.com

The author gratefully acknowledges the editing and proofreading assistance provided by Christine Michelle Davis, Shaylee Davis, Mariah Murphy, and Christine Shoaff-Brown.

The Silent Tongue (aphasia)

The words you do not hear the tears you cannot see
Are hidden within my nucleus, this is my new identity.
I am alike dry earth, shriveled and worn
With no nurturing to the soul
And I am quite helpless, in my world no longer whole.
So bear with me and try to creep inside this silent tent
My ills have bereaved my spirit
My soul is discontent.

Please do not look at me ... as if I am not here
Please do not speak to me ... as if I cannot hear.
Although I can't express myself with this muted speech of mine
My needs are very important it's difficult to define.
Please be polite and patient ... maintain my dignity
My mind is tired and weary with this disability.
I sit in silence in my room I cannot say "Good Morning Sun."
The words are tangled in my mind
Like twisted branches on a vine.

Those who speak in silence have a fervor.
We ... Who talk so freely don't understand or know.
Take a walk into a garden, see the flowers row on row
Their colors are bright, their life is sweet
And we hear words of passion in the silent way they speak.

Kathleen Gerety, RN
Atkinson, New Hampshire

Reflections on Global Aphasia

It came on suddenly. The stroke hit me like a club to the head wielded by the devil himself. The headache, blurred vision, and weakness literally brought me to my knees. Words failed me as I tried to explain to my wife and daughter the confusion and fear I felt. At first, the restaurant talk and clatter were unbearable, and then the silence and stares simply embarrassing. I felt the cold hand of death on my shoulder and I knew this place was where my life would end. All that was me in this world would end in this eating house after rhubarb cherry pie and coffee. It was so unreal.

I had beaten the odds of living three score and ten. Well into my eighties, my life had certainly lived up to the hype. Sometimes exciting and rarely boring, it had been a great adventure full of highs and lows, and many days of just "middlin" along. Until that day in the restaurant, I had met most of life's challenges with determination and some degree of competence, and frankly, I was proud of my track record. Yet nothing had prepared me for this stroke and the communication disorder known as "global aphasia." It appeared that my last life challenge was going to be the biggest one yet, for global aphasia is a nasty double-edged sword. It ravaged my life, and at the same time, took from me the tools to deal with it. But by far, the most brutal aspect of global aphasia was the collapse of the well-worn bridge of communication connecting me and my loved ones.

I have absolutely no recollection of the ambulance ride to the hospital or the stint in the emergency room. Neither do I remember the brain scans, punctured veins, catheter insertion, or other medical indignities I suffered that day. Looking back, my complete amnesia for the terrible events happening to me was, at least partially, a result of repression. That day was so traumatic I have blocked all memory of it. Welcome to the first day of the rest of my life as a global aphasic.

Don't get me wrong, I have never been a man to cower in desperate situations. I am not the kind of person to run and hide when the going gets tough. I have always risen to the occasion and prided myself on being a hard worker. I suppose the time I spent in the military taught me how to find the courage to meet hard challenges, but my youth spent on a farm laid the foundation for the mettle needed to survive global aphasia. It seems the first twenty years of one's life sets the character foundation for the scores to follow.

I remember opening my eyes and feeling the stiff sheets of my hospital bed. The intensive care unit was cold, dim, and sterile. The ceiling had those acoustic tiles with thousands of little holes to trap the sounds of pain and anguish. I lay on my back listening to the not-so-familiar hospital sounds. By the looks of the instruments attached to me, this appeared to be a very serious place. Humming sounds emanating from a blue machine with colorful graphs that showed the actions of my apparently still beating heart. There was a click, click, click of another expensive machine and the drone of several others jammed into the tiny space. The first inkling I had that all was not right with my brain was that these sounds seemed unusual and out-of-context. It was like I had never heard them before. Upon that realization, I felt my first tingling of anxiety and the need to escape this hell-hole.

My brain-damaged perception of those instruments reminded me of a haybaler, a farming machine with which I have much familiarity. I have spent many days, sunup to sundown, sitting on a huge tractor baling hay. From the time my father deemed me old enough to safely control a tractor, I rose at 4:00 a.m., ate a quick breakfast, and drove a farm pickup to the hay field with its miles of neatly cut rows of alfalfa. If the rows were sufficiently dry and aged, I would start the diesel tractor and let it warm up. As the sun peeked over the horizon to the fresh smell of green, I would engage the power-take-off, starting a large flywheel spinning on the baler. The increasing whir of the flywheel spinning faster was in sharp contrast to the lowered pitch of the tractor engine, as more power was needed to spin it. The baler conveyer would start to revolve, with small prongs slowly lifting the row of alfalfa for chomping by a mechanical jaw. The tractor, in one of the slowest creeping gears, would crawl along, rocking to the music of the haybaler. In front of the slow-moving baler was the cut alfalfa, and behind it, neat rows of 100 pound hay bales. Even today, the sounds emanating from that baler are as familiar to me as birds chirping and popcorn popping: low pitch tractor groans, spinning flywheel, crunching hay, and then every-so-often, the sound of mechanical arms tying thick twine into perfect square-knots. Concluding the baling symphony would be the final thud of a completed bale of hay dropping to the ground. As I lay on my back, staring at the acoustic tiles in that hospital room, my brain processed the hospital noise as those familiar farming sounds of my distant youth.

On some level, I knew that hay baling was not likely to be a function of the intensive care unit of this hospital, but that did not stop the disturbing auditory perceptions. Then, I heard the distinct knell of a telephone at the nurses' station and thought someone was knocking at my door. The unusual hospital sounds troubled me, but not nearly as much as the nurse's inquiry: "How are you doing?" She was a pleasant-looking person, about 30 years-old, with a fresh face and piercing blue eyes. To me however, I thought it only a courtesy that the hospital should hire an English speaking health care professional who would be polite enough not to mumble. Convinced that she was commenting on the unusual sounds emanating from the room, I tried to joke that apparently some farmer was baling hay in an adjacent room. She fluffed my pillow, checked the machines for aberrant sounds, and left the room.

Awakening that day into the world of global aphasia was, to say the least, disturbing. I knew something was awry mentally and physically. Though my eyes, skin, and nose were working well enough, my ears and mouth were haywire. I seemed alone in some unreal netherworld. To make matters worse, the right side of my body appeared dead. From the tips of my toes to the top of my head, the muscles on the right side of my body seemed broken and in need of repair. I tried to get up to escape this frightening twilight zone episode, but cloth restraints held me tightly to the hospital bed. Several times I attempted to shout to the fresh-faced nurse to help me, but I could not seem to remember the words, nor could I get my mouth to work properly. I couldn't even get my vocal cords to vibrate. Finally, I laid back and simply escaped the reality of my predicament. In the sanctuary of fantasy, I returned to comforting images of my past and mentally left the hospital room behind me. I found myself plowing a hay field. It was late afternoon, birds were chirping, a cool breeze flowed from the west, and for a brief time, all was right with my world.

The field being plowed was a quarter mile long. It was familiar and comforting. I dropped the six-point plow into the cut hayfield, pulled the tractor throttle completely back, and watched the black diesel exhaust fill the sky. The front wheel of the tractor dropped into the previously plowed groove and for the next fifteen minutes, the tractor tugged the plow blades deeply through the soil to the end of the row. As I lay on that hospital bed on that awful day, I returned to that field and I was once again young and healthy. I watched the birds, mostly gulls, soar above the turned soil looking for worms, mice, and grasshoppers. They glided so easily, often just out of my reach, eyes carefully scanning the freshly plowed field for a quick meal. Sometimes, they dropped to the ground, and briefly fought over an unfortunate creature. Eventually, one would win the treat and fly off with the prize with other birds in hot pursuit. On those crisp days of early spring, I dreamed the dreams of youth and possibilities. Only occasionally would I return to the hospital bed and to global aphasia, realizing that my future was now behind me.

In the intensive care unit, I had several visitors. Doctors, nurses, and lab technicians came and went. They greeted me in some foreign language, did their things, and left uttering farewells that were completely incomprehensible to me. Sometimes, I attempted a comment, but to no avail. Try as I may, my speech machine would not construct sounds, syllables, words, or phrases. The visitors seemed unconcerned about my lack of speech and apparently knew that the stroke had taken this part of my life. To them, global aphasia was no big deal and little pressure was placed on me to speak. It was the first visit from my wife and daughter that drove home the undeniable fact that global aphasia is indeed one big deal.

Although I could not tell whether it was morning or night in the artificially lit room, I saw them both enter. Forced smiles replaced grim expressions on their faces as they approached my bed. There stood my beautiful wife of more than a half-century and my precious daughter and mother of my grandchildren. Though language failed to organize my thoughts, there was no confusion about what an important part of my life they had always been. Love transcends the absence of language. My wife softly caressed my cheek and my daughter held my hand. Then, as though a flood gate had been abruptly opened, tears flowed from my eyes and I sobbed like a baby. This unexpected and uncontrolled outburst, far greater than the emotions I felt, dealt my self-esteem a devastating blow. Here, in front of my wife and daughter, I, a vigorous husband and strong-loving father, lie in a hospital bed crying like a baby. It was then that I had the first realization that life had dealt me one hell of a bad hand with this global aphasia. To add insult to brain injury, I could not explain to them that the crying was far out of proportion to the actual emotions I felt. Try as I may, I could not stop the crying. The embarrassment I felt was incredible. The fresh-faced nurse entered the room and uttered something unintelligible to me, but apparently meaningful to them, about "emotional lability." Call it what you want, but for me, it laid waste to my self-concept. I hated the speechless baby within me. I did not realize it that day, but global aphasia was to hit me with many more blows to my fragile self-esteem. The worst of them happened that evening.

That evening, as I stared at the muted television, I felt the familiar need to go to the bathroom. Looking around the room, I saw the bathroom door and tried to get up, but restraints and paralysis prevent movement. I started to feel panicky as the need to use the toilet rose. What to do? Realizing that I could not get to the bathroom myself, I tried to call for a nurse or an aide. Try as I may, I could not remember the words I needed to speak. Once, in my mind, I remembered the word "bathroom," or something like it, but programming my speech muscles to produce it was futile. I could not recollect how to get my lungs, voice box, and tongue to make the sounds. To make matters worse, every attempt to speak was met with resistance from paralyzed speech muscles. Desperately, I tried to get my good hand to push the blue call-button, but that too was beyond my abilities. I was not confused about these basic actions; I was perplexed. I knew what I needed to do, but I could not perform the simple speech and physical acts necessary to get them done.

Well, I am not going to go into detail about the events that followed, but suffice it to say, it was one of the most awful experiences I have suffered in my eighty-plus years on this planet. Thank God for a kind nurses' aide who cleaned me and the mess. When it was over, I lay in that bed with my once proud self-concept destroyed. Global aphasia had reduced me to a crying, incontinent, speechless baby. That day, I started the long slide into the deep, dark cavern of despair. I felt hopeless and helpless, and began wrestling with what the doctors call "clinical depression." I soon became painfully aware that depression in stroke survivors is often accompanied by anxiety. It was like having a depressing, dark cloud of dread hanging over my head causing near-unbearable anxiety and fear. On several occasions, I thanked God that suicide was at least one option for ending the pain.

I know doctors debate whether depression-anxiety is a reaction to stressful events or simply the result of brain chemicals gone awry. I also know that it really did not matter to me what caused my depression-anxiety. I suffered the angst, the despair and anxiety, for far too long before my handlers recognized my pain and rescued me from it. I am certain the stroke stirred up my brain chemistry, probably causing "feel good" chemicals to be in short supply. I also know that finding oneself in the world of global aphasia is one depressing realization. Fortunately, with the help of an antidepressant, counseling, love, and therapies, for the most part, my angst lifted. Remarkably, I found reasons to go on living as a global aphasic.

I wonder if any human escapes this world without suffering depression. I have certainly been depressed, sometimes deeply so. I am not going to dwell on it, but the death of my father in a farming accident caused severe grieving depression. Farming is such a dangerous business, and wearing loose-fitting clothing around the spinning flywheel of a haybaler can be, and was, deadly. I remember hiding the overwhelming grief I felt from everyone, including myself. I tried to "man-up" about it, especially around my mother. I never really cried when dad died. Only the loss of my dog, "Yeller," gave me the opportunity to grieve openly.

I know naming a dog "Yeller," isn't exactly the most creative thing I have done, and it ranks right up there with calling my first horse, "Flicka." But the name fit that little dog with yellow spots. Yeller took a liking to me from the first day I found him wandering the corrals. He followed me everywhere and spent long summer days trotting behind me or riding in the bed of the pickup, having more fun than any dog has the right to have. I must have been a junior in high school when I was mowing hay and accidently cut off his legs. He had followed me on every round that day, and on the last swath, I cut him down. He had chased a mouse or rabbit into the last row of alfalfa. I got off the tractor, nearly vomited, and yes, I cried like a baby and did so for most of that day. It was about a year after my father's death, and it prompted a year of grieving depression. I guess I had been repressing my father's death, and losing my dog opened the flood gates. Strangely, I felt comfortable crying over Yeller. It was something I could never do over the loss of my dad, since I was now the man of the house.

Eventually, I was transferred to the rehabilitation wing of the hospital. I'll never forget my first public entry into the real world as I was wheeled from one side of the hospital complex to the other. I sat in a wheelchair in my jogging clothes, my hair mussed, while an aide, whistling a silly tune, took me on my first journey as a disabled person. Moving through the halls, I saw busy nurses, doctors, and other health care workers pass me, clearly caught up in their own worlds. They were talking, sometimes laughing, and I suspected I was the butt of their jokes. I must have looked quite a sight. Several times, I tried to speak to the aide, but all that came from my paralyzed mouth was "tula, uh tula, tula." When words failed me, I attempted a smile only to produce a lopsided one with drool dripping from my mouth. I wished my handlers would have better dressed me, combed my hair, and made me as presentable as possible for this unveiling into the real world. For a moment during that journey, my depression was displaced by anger. I was angry at my handlers for neglecting my appearance, the aide for her indifference to my plight, the nurses, doctors, and other health care workers for laughing at me, and at God for causing this disaster in the first place.

Global aphasia put a strain on my relationship with God. The devil stroke took prayer and the intimate words I always shared with my creator. From the time I was a child in Sunday school, my belief in God had been my joy and comfort. I know what you must be thinking, that I am some religious fanatic clinging to some outdated organized religion because of fear and ignorance. Maybe there is some truth to that, but then, so what? It might surprise you to know that my belief in God has evolved over the years. As a child, and like all children, I personified God as a kind man living above me, directing my life, and protecting me. I found wise counsel in God during my formative years. As a teenager, I rebelled, and for a short time, I believed in nothingness, randomness, and chance. Intellectually, I just could not accept the divine story, but it was a very unsatisfying existence for me.

As a young adult, I returned to some of my beliefs, and with education and life-experiences, I conceptualized God as more of an abstraction. In my later years, I still felt an invisible presence of something grand in the universe. Much of my religious philosophy was thought out during day-long tractor work. It radiated from within and without me and did not need defining or description. Before the stroke, I had managed to be at peace with my consciousness as simply a property of matter, evolving from the glorious "Big Bang" to that which is me. I had a belief in a greater, ordered scheme of things. Remarkably, I was able to reconcile my evolved belief with my early religious teachings and they fit together nicely. Throughout my years of living, even during my atheist period, I have always been one to pray silently, not just during difficult times, but to put into language my awe and joy of life. Global aphasia took the spiritual words from me and I experienced a deep sense of abandonment and isolation. Fortunately, as time passed, I learned that God is greater than a small clogged blood vessel in my brain and this devilish global aphasia.

My speech-language pathologist has been a big part of my post-stroke life. She is much younger than me, as are most people nowadays. She knew enough not to be to bubbly or overly optimistic, yet neither was she a pessimist or a hard realist. She was competent and knowledgeable about this damnable global aphasia. However, we did get off to a rocky start during the initial evaluation session. Her need to know the details of my global aphasia was in conflict with my difficulties adjusting to it.

The therapy suite was brightly and tastefully decorated, neither too large nor small. A window looked out into a grove of oak trees with colorful leaves falling to the ground. She sat behind a small wooden table and I faced her. She laid out several pictures and objects on the table and proceeded to ask me questions: "Point to the fork," "Fill in the blank," Write this," "Repeat that," "Read this sentence," and "Tell me this, that, and the other thing." She carefully took notes on my accomplishments, or more often, on my confusion and verbal impotence. I know she was merely trying to find out what the stroke had taken from my once normal ability to communicate, but it was the first time I had been confronted with the entirety of my global aphasia. By the time the evaluation was completed, I was shaken to the core. My previously easy and second-nature communication acts were now a thing of the past. Oh, she was pleasant enough and several times she allowed me to compose myself. Nevertheless, on that day, I was subjected to the totality of what the stroke hath wrought. I was told I would have "trial therapy" to see what I could regain in the realm of communication.

The next day, I began my therapy regimens, which would continue for weeks. Usually, my handlers awakened me at 7:00 a.m. and I was taken to the communal dining room. There, with the assistance of an aide, I was fed a pureed breakfast. Eating took much longer than before the stroke because I had difficulty managing and swallowing the stuff. After breakfast, and after the food remnants were cleaned from my face, I was taken to the physical therapy gym where I usually failed at standing on my own, transferring from wheelchair to real chair, and keeping my balance. An occupational therapist watched me fail at most activities of daily living, which previously I had done without a second thought. I had morning and afternoon sessions with the speech-language pathologist and it was during one of them that I had my first frightening panic attack.

My speech-language pathologist was showing me large pictures of common objects: a house, car, and cow. She, by word and deed, asked me to supply the name to each picture. First, she lifted the picture of the house from the table and placed in it front of me. I recognized it for what it was. For heaven's sake, I knew what a house was! Yet for the life of me, I could not recall the name. My mind was a blank. Then, she showed me the car. Again, I knew it was a car, but I sat there in silence. I tried and tried to recall the word, worked to make my mouth properly move, but it was to no avail. I had the depressing realization for the first time that there was something seriously wrong with my mind, and the anxiety grew. I was not in control of my own body.

The room began to get smaller and smaller, and I started to sweat. I could hardly catch my breath. On a nonverbal level, I admitted to myself that I could not even come up with these simple names—something a small child could do with ease. When she showed me the picture of a cow, I felt the need to escape, to get out of the room and all it threatened. I felt trapped and isolated from the rest of the world. I panicked when I recognized not only that it was a cow, but a Holstein milker, a type of dairy cow I spent many mornings and evenings milking. Many like it had been a large part of my life, yet I was incapable of even saying the word, "cow." What had become of my mind? I pushed the picture away and tried to wheel myself from the therapy suite. I needed to get out of there. Fortunately, the speech-language pathologist recognized my reaction to this self-concept catastrophe, and removed the pictures from the table. We took a break from the trauma. She talked in a soothing voice about something or other, pointed to the colorful oak tree, and after a while, I regained my composure.

The weeks in rehabilitation were the most intense days of my long life. Physical and occupational therapies were challenging, but the drills and exercises to regain my ability to communicate were by far the most distressing. With physical and occupational therapies, I worked on tangible aspects of my life taken by the stroke such as walking, eating, and dressing myself. The goals of physical and occupational therapies were things I could see and touch; they were practical and concrete. However, the therapies to regain my speech and language involved many intangible and often elusive goals. We worked on my thoughts, expressions, and understanding of other people's statements. Exercises dealing with reading, writing, and gesturing were more tangible because I could at least see the results of my efforts, meager though they were.

Every day in rehabilitation, I was confronted with my physical and mental limitations, which taxed my ability to cope with all that had been taken from me. Fortunately, my depression and anxiety were lifting due to the antidepressant and the love and support from all involved in my new life as a stroke survivor. Unfortunately, I was not making significant gains in any of the therapies. After several weeks, my handlers determined it was in my best interest to be sent home. There was discussion about a nursing home, but my wife and daughter said that with the help from home health nurses and therapists, I could likely spend the rest of my days at home. At least they would give it a try.

I think the most distressing thing about global aphasia was that I was left out of the decision process about how my life would continue. It was a troubling yet necessary aspect of global aphasia. Due to my inability to communicate, I simply had to rely on the kindness of strangers and the love and support of my wife and daughter. The last thing I wanted was to be a burden, especially to my loved ones.

I am pleasantly surprised to find that there is life after global aphasia. It has been nearly a year since I fell to my knees in that restaurant knocking the rhubarb cherry pie to the floor. Now, as I sit here in my back yard watching bluebirds eat from the feeder, I have some sense of the meaning of it all. I seem to have reached an acceptance of my situation, and I feel neither good nor bad about it. It is just the way things have worked out for me. Like an early-autumn killing frost, global aphasia has been an unwanted intrusion into the sunset of my life. Yet this communication disorder has not destroyed the seeds I have sown or the rich harvest of my experiences. As I stare at the sun setting over the horizon and savor the magnificent autumn colors of my beloved farm, I bask in what has been rather than what has been lost. Global aphasia, formidable though it may be, is but one of my life experiences, seeded with challenges, but also carrying the promise of a plentiful harvest of growth, understanding, and acceptance.

A Trip to the Fire Station

The walk from my office to the group therapy suite is about the length of a football field. I enjoy the short jaunt through the halls of this busy hospital. Today, I see several nurses talking with animated gestures, eagerly discussing something of common interest. I greet a physical therapist and smile to a doctor as we pass each other. I glance into an administrative office, a vice president of something or other, and admire her lavish furnishings. I turn the corner and pass by the nurses' station. I nod to a patient in a wheelchair parked next to it. She is a young woman with head bandages and her right arm in a sling. I see the door to my destination, and slowly open it. My four patients sit in wheelchairs facing a large conference table and I pull up my chair.

I smile and greet each of them with a pleasant, "Good morning," "Nice to see you," and "Hello." I comment that it is a fine morning, and suggest we get down to work.

"Can anyone name this object?" I ask.

I search the faces of the four patients sitting in front of me for any indication of a desire to respond to my query.

"You write with it," I say, offering the cue and demonstrating writing on a sheet of imaginary paper.

Still no response. Resigned that this will likely be a long hour, I hold a key before them and ask, "What is this called?" I rotate it several times to show its function, but still no reply.

I decide to ask each patient individually to respond and begin with Mrs. Johnson. She should be the most likely to participate, given her intact language abilities. Barbara Johnson suffers from amyotrophic lateral sclerosis and we are working on speech intelligibility. There is no question that she knows the name of the objects, but today, she appears too unmotivated to reply to my question.

Barbara is 38 years old and has been in steady decline for the past three months. I know there are no good diseases, but ALS, Lou Gehrig's disease, is such a bad one. During the initial evaluation, she told me the first sign of it was chronic fatigue. Now, of course, every day I feel tired, I suspect my upper and lower motor neurons are starting to degenerate.

Barbara has two young children and her marriage is failing. Her husband takes care of the kids, but rarely visits her. Their marriage was in trouble long before the onset of the disease, and now she knows there is no hope of salvaging it. At least she can take solace in knowing their father will care for the children after she is gone. The average survival time for ALS patients is three years.

I hold the picture of the key to her again and prompt: "Try to say this as clearly as possible, Barbara."

This time she utters an unvoiced connection of nasalized vowels, bearing no resemblance to the word.

"Nice try," I say, and encourage her to valve the /k/ phoneme more clearly. She wipes the drool from her mouth. I turn to Lou and ask him to help Barbara say the word.

About 14 months ago, Lou DeRosa was diagnosed with a malignant brain tumor in the left hemisphere of his brain. The rumor floating around the hospital is that the only symptoms he had of the large tumor were headaches and numbness in his right hand. Yesterday, I too had a headache and wondered if I had a cancerous brain tumor eating away at my gray matter.

After a brief delay, Lou clearly says the word, "key," and I automatically give him the nonverbal prompt, an expansion of my hands, to lengthen the utterance.

He dutifully says, "That is she, uh, key."

"Great expansion, Lou," I say, and give him the thumbs-up gesture.

Seeing that Lane, a traumatic brain injured patient, is distracted and leaning over the left side of his wheelchair, I try to bring him into the group therapy session and recall the tragic car accident that caused his brain damage. He and a friend, another high school senior, were racing on the outskirts of town. A quarter-mile stretch of road had been marked with white paint, and on weekends, racers lined up and raced the distance in their muscle cars. One night, Lane, with his lifelong buddy sitting in the passenger seat, carefully situated the front tires of the 1967 Camaro Super Sport to the starting line. Next to them, another high school acquaintance similarly set his Japanese "rice burner" in position. The race was excitingly loud, and Lane handily won it as he sped past the finish line at nearly 100 miles-per-hour.

Then, his right front tire blew, and the restored Camaro flipped end-over-end, ejecting him and instantly killing his friend. Lane suffered a massive head injury. Now, this teenager who reveled in the thrill of speed and acceleration sits nearly motionless and is confined to a wheelchair. Lane has aphasia, dysarthria, and problems with mental executive control.

Getting Lane to pay attention during group has been challenging, to say the least. He is a confused and agitated Level IV on the *Rancho Los Amigos Scale*. I show him the key and he utters something unintelligible about a car ride to a fire station. Barbara and Lou make eye-contact with me and we share perplexed expressions. Then, I look to Ruth, the final member of our motley crew, to supply the name for the object. I know she is capable of attempting a response if she can navigate through her cloud of depression.

Ruth is a 57-year-old diabetic. She suffered the typical CVA which causes aphasia and apraxia of speech in so many of my patients. The occlusion was to the left middle cerebral artery, damaging Broca's and surrounding areas in the posterior inferior frontal lobe. She also has right hemiparesis. As often happens in many patients with predominantly expressive aphasia, she initially also had mild receptive language difficulties. However, her score on the recently administered *Token Test* showed she can now understand most of the speech of others. While she has apraxia of speech and difficulties programming utterances, the majority of her expressive problems involve anomia: word-finding problems. As I reported during the Tuesday morning rehabilitation meeting, Ruth has "Broca's aphasia with a preponderance of anomia."

As also happens with the majority of patients with this type of brain injury, she is clinically depressed and anxious. She was prescribed an antidepressant, but it has not had time to combat her depression-anxiety.

Ruth is unable to recall the name of the object and appears more depressed than usual. I pat her knee, and say, "Nice try."

Apparently, Lou has something important to say to the group. He starts by saying, "Don't you know, don't you know, the sit, sit, it is sit, in head."

All but Lane turn to Lou in anticipation of this announcement of something profound. Again, he says in earnest, "Don't you know. The sit is in the sit. Now, tell me."

Barbara looks to me for interpretation. Lou again tells the group of the "sit," and asks us, "Don't you know?"

Tension builds in the room and Ruth begins to cry. I comfort Ruth while trying to decipher Lou's important statement. I decide to use this increase in group energy to prompt more interaction and communication.

"Lou," I say, "Try one word at a time."

This time, with firm resolve, he says carefully, "The sit, don't . . . you . . . know."

Ruth's crying subsides as Lane takes center stage again with the announcement that last night, nurses apparently loaded him into a car and drove him to a nearby fire station.

Barbara, Lou, and Ruth now give Lane their undivided attention. I wonder how prudent it is to have the entire group's attention focused on Lane's delusional trip to a fire station. I know it would be extremely unlikely for nurses to take Lane from his room, load him in a car, and drive him anywhere. I glance at his chart and see "posttraumatic psychosis" on the cover sheet.

Barbara takes the lead for the group and asks Lane, "What are you talking about?"

Actually, she produced a series of hypernasal vowels and indistinct consonants, but it was intelligible enough to be understood by most of the group.

Lou offers a follow-up question: "The sit station?"

Now Ruth shows interest in Lane's response, and comments: "Sire, shire, kire house?"

Lane, with even more resolve, but with apparent tolerance for the group's incredulity, relates the late night trip to a fire station apparently as some kind of reward for his good behavior. I decide to confront Lane with his irrationality, and open his chart to the nursing section. Given Lane's mental and physical status, I needed to confirm my suspicion that this was indeed a delusional field trip. As I suspected, there was no reference to a trip to a fire station. As I closed the chart, I see a nurse's note alluding to Lane's reward for good behavior. Last night, he was allowed to sit next to the nurses' station and watch the goings-on from that vantage point. Not only did he not leave the facility last night, he spent much of it under the careful scrutiny of several nurses. I have seen patients bask in that special privilege with their wheelchairs parked next to the large glass-enclosed fire hose beside the nurses' station.

Lou, with urgency in his voice, comments on Lane's announcement: "The sit, the sit, don't . . . you . . . know."

He seems to understand what Lane is saying. Then, Lou gestures to the door of the room, points to Lane and says, "He sit, sit, nurse."

I decide things are getting out-of-hand in group today. Now, it appears that Lou is sharing a delusional trip to a fire station with Lane. For a moment, I entertain the idea of going to the fire station and asking the firefighters if our residents visited them last night.

I decide to do more naming exercises and address word-finding paraphasias. Most of the word-finding responses of my aphasic patients are verbal paraphasias, association errors, where they don't say the correct word, but one associated with it. "Pen" for "pencil" and "lock" for "key" are likely naming errors made by Lou, Ruth, and Lane. Lane! Association errors! Lane often produces verbal paraphasias during naming exercises. Then, I realize that the diagnosis of "posttraumatic psychosis" in Lane's chart may be greatly exaggerated, at least with respect to a delusional trip to a fire station.

Apparently, last evening, Lane was helped into his wheelchair and transported to the glass-enclosed fire hose by the nurses' station. He was placed in his car (wheelchair) and driven (wheeled) to the fire station (fire hose). Lane was not reporting a delusional trip; he was simply describing, using verbal paraphasias, the special privilege he was given the previous evening. Evidently, Lou witnessed the event and was trying to explain it to me. I explain to the group that I finally get it, and apologize for my misunderstanding. I am more than a little embarrassed by it all and wonder if I have receptive language problems. Then, I turn to Barbara and ask her to say as clearly as possible, "Fire hose," and to please do so emphasizing the consonants. Obviously relieved by the resolution of Lane's not-so-delusional trip to a fire station, she managed to produce the /f/ and /z/ in the words clearly.

"Great job," I say and remind her that these things are measured in small but important steps.

The rest of the session was uneventful. On my way back to my office, I pass by the nurses' station and again see the patient parked next to the glass-enclosed fire hose.

I say "Hello," not expecting a response, and none was forthcoming. I turn the corner and wonder if she will be diagnosed with posttraumatic psychosis.

The Reunion

The Grand Canyon is one of the most popular tourist destinations in the United States. Each year, thousands of tourists pass through Flagstaff, Arizona, and motor the hundred miles or so to the Grand Canyon National Park. An Irish couple, newlyweds on their honeymoon, was returning from this spectacular wonder of the natural world when they were involved in a serious automobile accident. Another car crossed the highway median, causing a head-on collision. Both newlyweds sustained closed head injuries and were transported to a regional head trauma center. The couple survived the accident, and after several weeks in a rehabilitation center, they were to be reunited. Tragically, the husband had virtually no memory of his marriage, honeymoon, or bride.

William and Bonnie married in Ireland, and immediately after the ceremony, traveled to New York City. From the Big Apple, they flew to Flagstaff where they rented a small gas-efficient car and drove to the Grand Canyon National Park. At the south rim of the Grand Canyon, they hiked the 10-mile trail down to the Colorado River and stayed at the rustic Phantom Ranch. They fished the Bright Angel Creek for Rainbow Trout and hiked the trails, marveling at the ancient beauty of it all. The young lovers remarked to each other that witnessing the Grand Canyon was the perfect start of their lives together. The next day, they returned to the top of the canyon, exhausted and sore. That evening, on the narrow road to Flagstaff, the automobile accident ended their future together. Eleven months later, they would sign divorce papers.

The therapists, doctors, and nurses of the rehabilitation center were concerned about the impending reunion of the newlywed couple. At the rehabilitation team meeting that morning, much time was spent discussing the reunion. Most of the team agreed that Bonnie's memories of events before the accident were returning nicely, and she would likely have near-complete recovery of cognitive functions. The neuropsychologist noted that few patients with posttraumatic amnesia ever regain all of their memory about the events surrounding the accident, and Bonnie would be no exception. However, Bonnie recalled much of her prior relationship with William and either remembered the events leading to the accident or learned about them from reports. The social worker observed that Bonnie was understandably anxious about the reunion. Yet the real concern for the rehabilitation team was about William and his reaction to seeing his bride for the first time since the accident.

According to the rehabilitation team neurologist, William suffered a severe closed head injury. He was unconscious at the scene for longer than thirty minutes and suffered nearly complete retrograde amnesia for events related to his wife, marriage, and honeymoon. The patient continued to be disorientated times four, i.e., time, place, person, and situation-predicament, and was undergoing reality orientation with few positive results. In addition, he was confused, angry, agitated, and socially disinhibited. The occupational therapist reported that William walked naked through the halls recently and occasionally struck out at others, especially when frustrated.

The newlywed reunion was scheduled for noon that day in the conference room. Earlier, the social worker prepared Bonnie for the cognitive and behavioral changes she might see in William, but reminded her that he was still recovering from the head injury and would likely improve. Bonnie came early and sat at the end of the long conference table, anxious about seeing her husband. She wore a white blouse and blue skirt, and had obviously spent much time on her appearance. Several rehabilitation center staff members entered the room, wished Bonnie the best, and assured her all would work out for them. Tension built throughout the rehabilitation center as the reunion approached.

The occupational therapist and an aide helped William into a wheelchair. While transferring from bed to wheelchair, William continually uttered nonsensical statements about the size of his room, delusional visits from family members, and rats floating in a river. When told he would be meeting his wife, Bonnie, he stopped talking, and for an instant, it appeared he understood what was forthcoming. Then, William placed his hand on the thigh of the aide and uttered a profanity. The aide admonished him for his inappropriate behavior, unlocked the wheelchair, and began the short trip to the conference room. On the elevator, a nurse joined them and William made a lewd remark and attempted to fondle her. As they moved through the hall toward to the conference room, William again uttered suggestive statements to several women passing by. Before entering the conference room, William was again told he would be seeing Bonnie, his wife, for the first time since the accident. However, he seemed not to register the significance of the impending reunion.

The aide wheeled William to the conference table facing Bonnie. After a few minutes of silence, William pushed the wheelchair back from the table, looked to the social worker, and uttered a nonsense statement about river rats. Yet, the deep structure of the nonsense statement was clear; William had no recollection of the woman sitting across from him. Bonnie reached for his hand and began to cry. She said she loved him and tried to caress his arm. William pulled back and indicated, in no uncertain terms, that he wanted to return to his room. Bonnie again expressed her love for him, but it was a one-sided gesture. William clearly did not want anything to do with the stranger sitting across from him.

Rehabilitation professionals witness many of life's dramas. However, that day, the sad reunion of the newlywed couple caused even the most seasoned of them to have a heavy heart. Of course, no one blamed William for his actions, or more importantly, his inactions. The reality of traumatic brain injury is that it can, and often does, profoundly alter the lives of those affected by it. The reunion of the newlywed couple that day was a tragic reminder of the dreadful, and often irreversible, implications of traumatic brain injury.

Cautious Clyde's Descent into Darkness

"Cautious Clyde's Descent into Darkness" was originally published in *The Psychology of Neurogenic Communication Disorders: A Primer for Health Care Professionals* (Pearson Allyn & Bacon Publishers).

Clyde felt more secure landing at Spring Valley Airport than at any other tower-operated airstrip in the state. It wasn't because Spring Valley was controlled better than other airports of its size, it was because the small airport had little traffic and the calm winds flowed north to south, the same way runway "one eight five" coursed. The surrounding pine-covered mountains left little to the demands of navigation. A pilot had to be blind to miss Spring Valley. The Sawtooth mountain range was to the north, Lake Mary to the east, and to the west was the burnt ridge. Lately, the green was returning to the ridge, golden wild flowers could be seen, and the underbrush was gaining a foothold on the steep, rocky slopes. The residents of Spring Valley never discussed the burnt ridge; they seemed to accept the blackened expanse of the fire's wrath with the same tolerance they displayed for the cold dry winters of the Rockies.

Clyde considered him self a good pilot, as do all pilots, but Clyde's record supported his belief. He'd never as much as scratched a wing of an airplane, never dented a fuselage. Of course, few living pilots have scratched a wing of an airplane or dented a fuselage. In aviation, minor mishaps are rare and the word "mishap" is a misnomer when labeling accidents in mid-air. You don't have mishaps—you have disasters. Clyde was ever cautious, sometimes too cautious, but he was a cautious pilot nonetheless. This flight was no exception. Rather than contacting the tower when he reached the highest peak of Sawtooth range, which was about five miles from the airstrip, Clyde insisted on contacting Spring Valley Tower a good ten miles from the airport traffic area. FAA rules were as clear as the bureaucrats could make them, and five miles was the minimum contact distance for incoming flights. Clyde was cautious all right; if five miles was safe, ten miles was safer.

"Spring Valley Tower, Cessna three four four five niner, ten miles north inbound for landing," Clyde hailed in his most relaxed pilot's voice. He could barely see the top of the tower from his ten-mile vantage point. The brown log-constructed buildings and the accompanying mile-long, paved runway was a welcome sight to many a lost pilot. The joy of finding the airport from the green expanse of pine trees was inversely proportional to the amount of fuel remaining in the airplane's fuel tanks.

A few seconds later, the tower responded to his hail. "Cessna three four four five niner, Spring Valley Tower. Left traffic, runway one eight five, winds one seven zero at five, gusts to fifteen, altimeter two zero zero eight. Report downwind. Your traffic is a Piper on final."

Clyde adjusted his dark glasses as he acknowledged the landing instructions into the microphone attached to the left muff of the Sony headset: "Cessna four five niner"

Eight hundred hours. Eight hundred and seventy-two hours to be exact. That was the time Clyde had logged in single-engine land aircraft. Those hours made for responding to airport instructions as second-nature as obeying the only traffic signal in downtown Spring Valley. Nicole, the tower operator and Clyde's friend of twenty years, simply wanted this blue Cessna with the white markings N34459, and the colorful hand-painted eagle on each side of the tail, to turn parallel to the runway and to keep a southerly heading. As per Nicole's request, Clyde contacted the tower when the parallel turn had been completed.

Gusts of wind up to fifteen knots were not a problem, especially when they coursed from the south. Crosswinds were occasionally a problem, but not here, and not today. It would be another safe landing. At least, that was what Clyde thought.

Clyde descended to 1,000 feet above the Ponderosa pines. He reduced the power to 2,000 RPMs and ten degrees of flaps slowed the descent. He heard a reduction in noise when he cut the power and the quiet reminded Clyde to lower the nose of the plane.

"Keep your nose down and your speed up" echoed the words of his first flight instructor.

On the next turn, the plane slowed even more as Clyde added another 10 degrees of flaps. Once again, he lowered the nose and pushed the hand-held throttle to increase his speed, and gave the tower a final notification of his intentions: "Cessna three four four five niner on final." A few seconds later, he heard Nicole's professional voice clear him for landing as he added the final adjustment to the plane's flaps.

Flying is boring. Well, a lot of the time it is boring. Once the airplane is in the air and vectored to its destination, there is little for the pilot to do. With an adjustment here and there, the plane automatically and obediently cuts the air to its destination. Takeoff is fun. There is that pleasant sensation as the airplane lifts from the confines of the runway to the freedom of the sky. But landing the airplane is the biggest challenge of all. So much to do, so much to know, so many things that can go wrong. The landing strip seems small and approaches too fast. Worst of all, you are "low," "slow," and "heavy," with little time and few options if something goes wrong. And that day, for Clyde, something went terribly wrong.

About a football field from touchdown, a gust of wind blew his Cessna to the ground. There was no warning, no advanced notice. The down gust of wind simply caused the plane to drop like a rock to the pavement below. Clyde had little time to react. As per training and experience, he applied full throttle to gain speed. But it was too little, too late, and he was too low to the ground.

Just before the Cessna hit the ground, Clyde pulled back on the yoke and braced himself. These were reflex reactions as was his denial. He didn't believe what was happening; airplane crashes always happened to the other guy. This time, he was the other guy. On impact, the right wheel strut broke, causing the airplane to tip to the right while the nose and wing dug into the pavement. The propeller bent and abruptly stopped. Clyde felt the seat belt and shoulder harness cut into his waist and shoulders as he was thrown forward. Then the blue Cessna with the white markings N34459, and the colorful hand-painted eagle on each side of the tail, simply flipped over and slid to a halt on the asphalt.

The impact caused the fuselage to crush like paper. The engine of the airplane broke from its mounts and pushed back into the cockpit, and in doing so, broke both of Clyde's legs. The pain was unbearable. The top of the cabin of the airplane collapsed on impact, and Clyde's head slammed into the instrument panel. The plane skidded to a halt, sparks flying and smoke rising. Clyde's last thought was of the high test fuel in the wing tanks of the airplane, and the explosion he hoped was not inevitable.

Nicole watched Clyde's final descent to the airport. She never tired of the grace and beauty of an airplane, no matter how small, in its careful, controlled transformation from an air machine to a ground one. She thought of Clyde carefully and skillfully controlling the flying machine. When she saw the Cessna hit the pavement, flip, and skid, for an instant she did not believe her eyes. When the disaster finally registered in her mind, she automatically hit the large, red button on her control panel, which sounded the emergency alert. She had never pushed the red button for real, outside the monthly routine tests, and it surprised her how loud the siren was, and how it disrupted the morning calm.

The "wherrrrr, wherrrrr, wherrrrr" of the emergency siren sent two red trucks to the crumpled Cessna. The larger red truck sprayed chemicals on the smoldering airplane. A man dressed in a bright yellow spacesuit jumped from the smaller truck and ran to the pilot's aid. Clyde hung from his seat belt and shoulder harness, blood flowing from his head. He was unstrapped and pulled a safe distance from the smoking wreck. Soon, an ambulance from Spring Valley Hospital arrived, secured him to a gurney, and rushed Clyde to the only hospital in the county.

Eventually, the Cessna was completely drenched in chemicals. Thanks to God, luck, or the aeronautical engineers at the Cessna plant, the fuel in the wing tanks did not explode. Other airplanes were diverted to nearby airports, and the ones short of fuel were allowed to land on the narrow taxi strip.

As regulations required, Nicole notified the National Transportation Safety Board (NTSB) and an investigator was sent to determine the cause of the crash. Somehow, determining the cause of the crash seemed to bring closure to it. Of course, the cause would be "pilot error." It seemed it was always the pilot's fault. If the wings of an airplane are struck by lightning and blown to bits, it would be pilot error. In the view of the NTSB, a non-errant pilot would dodge the lightning. Ultimately, it was determined that Clyde, cautious Clyde, was too slow and too low for the weather conditions. The down gust of wind and the crash could have been avoided by a better pilot, a safer one.

Clyde did not register the months that passed since the crash of the Cessna. The passage of time for a person in a coma has often been compared to sleeping. It is not. The biggest difference between sleep and coma is that a sleeping person can be awakened. People in a coma also sleep. But nothing could awaken Clyde during those months. Not pain, hunger, the shouted words from his family and his friend, Nicole. For Clyde, those months were full of darkness. He would just as well have been in oblivion. There was no awareness of him self or the expensive hospital room that had become his home. There was no passage of time for Clyde. From the last, frightening images of the airplane crash to the sounds and blurry images he experienced months later, Clyde was in limbo. It was like he was on automatic pilot.

The formal diagnosis on Clyde's chart was "traumatic brain injury—closed." This simply meant that during the crash of the Cessna, his head slammed into the instrument panel, damaging and killing brain cells. The massive amounts of blood covering him and the cockpit of the airplane came from his head, but only the surface areas. There was no penetration into his brain, but even minor head wounds bleed profusely. Initially, there was a buildup of blood inside his brain. The broken blood vessels spilled their contents into his head, and with nowhere to go, the pressure continued to rise, posing a risk of death. Apparently, if the pressure within the skull becomes greater than the heart's ability to circulate the blood in the brain, then brain death can occur. Fortunately, a skilled brain surgeon (Are there unskilled brain surgeons?) put a tube in his brain to drain the fluid and release the pressure, ultimately saving Clyde's life.

Believe it or not, one of the biggest medical complications was bed sores. For some reason, Clyde was not turned, rolled and moved enough to prevent them. The worst one was at the base of his spine. Once it started, it got bigger and bigger. Eventually, salve, light and medication helped, but the bed sores became a serious problem. For a while, Clyde was put in a bed that blew small, round pellets around inside the mattress. Had

Clyde been aware of what was happening, he would have had the sensation of floating in air.

In flight training, instructors talk about losing and regaining orientation. In darkness, it is easy to become disoriented. Sometimes, when it is very dark and the sky is overcast, a pilot can become disoriented so as to lose ground reference. This means that the pilot might confuse the ground for the sky because the balance centers in the inner ear can be confused as well. Because of an airplane's rapid turn, it can give the pilot a sense of a normal flight path when, in fact, the airplane might be in a steep dive. Of course, the instrument panel can provide valuable information about climbing, turning, and speed. Tragically, some pilots panic, do not believe their instruments, and a disaster is the result. As Clyde gradually came out of his coma, he too was disoriented, not just to his environment, but to time, people, and situations as well. Unfortunately, there was no instrument panel to guide him through the mental cloud.

When Clyde's head hit the Cessna's instrument panel, the impact damaged his brain, resulting in memory problems, disorientation, and higher level language deficits. Combined, these problems caused Clyde to act in strange ways. The disorientation experienced by a pilot in darkness is similar to that experienced by head trauma patient. For the pilot, disorientation occurs when the demands of the environment exceed his or her knowledge and experience. For Clyde, the mental disorientation he experienced was also due to the interplay between the environment and his cognitive status. The environmental demands exceeded his abilities.

Late one afternoon, Nicole stopped by the hospital to visit Clyde, her friend of twenty years. He had moved from the intensive care unit to intermediate care, a step down unit. Although he was no longer unconscious, his words and actions were bizarre. It was apparent he did not know where he was or what had happened to him.

Clyde was sitting in a large chair with a table attached to it. To prevent him from escaping or falling over, a tied sheet held him in an upright position. His room was small and the walls were plastered with large-print calendars, pictures of family members, and a blackboard with his daily schedule written in yellow chalk. As Nicole entered the room, the unmistakable odor of a sweaty male was almost overwhelming. But what was indeed overwhelming was what Clyde did next.

As Nicole saw Clyde, she immediately felt a wave of sorrow flood over her. She walked across the room to give him a friendly, supportive hug and he did something normal Clyde would never do. He grasped her breast and said, in slurred speech that made it all the more vulgar, the most offensive thing Nicole had ever heard. Startled, Nicole stepped back and tried to comprehend how Clyde could have been transformed into the monster in the chair, and again, he uttered the offensive statement with a wild, profane look on his face. Shocked, Nicole left the room, almost in tears. She needed to get away from what he had become. A nurse saw the startled look on her face and suggested they go to the lounge for a cup of coffee. Nicole consented, hopeful that the nurse could explain what had happened to her friend of twenty years.

The kind nurse explained that Clyde was not responsible for his behavior because he had impaired executive functioning. The brain injury he suffered removed regulatory functions from his personality. With no sense of appropriate or inappropriate, Clyde's normal and natural urges had free reign to control his actions. Clyde's normal sexual urges and needs were not regulated, and his actions were a result of this change in his personality. Nicole began to understand that Clyde's behaviors would gradually become more appropriate as he improved, and there was a good likelihood that he would once again be the gentle, polite person she befriended twenty years ago. Sadly, it was unlikely Clyde would return to complete normalcy. People who suffer serious brain injuries rarely make complete recovery. But, Nicole learned that Clyde would likely recover many of his thought processes and physical abilities. After the meeting with the nurse, Nicole was optimistic about Clyde's potential. Most importantly, she understood that much of what he was going through was a temporary, and necessary, part of the recovery from a closed head-injury.

Just as the kind nurse predicted, over the next few months Clyde improved considerably. His broken legs healed and some movement returned to his arm. Clyde's memory was still defective, especially for new information, but he was able to manage day-to-day activities. He gradually remembered faces and people from his life before the crash of the Cessna. Ultimately, he was able to live relatively independently in a group home not far from the airport, where so many months ago, he began his descent into darkness.

Crossed Aphasia in a Dextral:
The Brain Localization Debate

The results of the evaluation were unequivocal. The patient, Ruth Lamb, clearly suffered from "crossed aphasia," "nondominant aphasia," or the more clinically correct diagnosis of "crossed aphasia in a dextral." All brain scans showed the infarction to be in the right hemisphere, particularly the precentral gyrus, yet the test results showed severe Broca's aphasia and left hemiparalysis.

Good friends for many years, the aphasiologist and the neuropsychologist discussed the case over coffee in the hospital dining room late one Saturday morning. Although their friendship had endured professional differences throughout the years, nothing taxed it more than the brain localization controversy, particularly concerning language. The aphasiologist believed the brain operates holistically with regard to phonology, grammar, and semantics, and the neuropsychologist was convinced that there are language centers, modules, of the brain.

Some consider the neuropsychologist to be an associationist and the aphasiologist a cognitivist. Associationists believe language is simply a labeling system and that a person's intelligence is located outside the major so-called language centers of the brain. According to the association theory, aphasia is a disturbance labeling objects, events, and ideas and can be attributed to specific damaged cortical areas of the brain. Cognitivists, on the other hand, challenge the idea that language is simply a labeling system in adults. They believe language and thought are integrally related and are a function of the brain operating as a whole. According to the cognitive theory, aphasia is a fundamental impairment in verbal symbolic processing and not merely a labeling disorder resulting from focalized lesions. Although certain areas of the brain are important for language, no single area can be considered a language center operating independently of other parts of the brain.

Regardless of the labels given to them, the aphasiologist and neuropsychologist felt strongly about their positions on localizing human brain function. At first, they sat alone in the dining room, but toward the end of the hour-long discussion, several health care professionals had joined them at the table to witness the impromptu debate. As one observer remarked at the end of the hotly-contested hour, it was one of the best in-service programs she had ever attended.

Ruth resided in Sedona, Arizona, a small town noted for its spectacular red rock formations and a population of retired actors, artists and the wealthy. The 62-year-old patient had no personal history of left-handedness nor did any of her immediate family. She was dining at an upscale restaurant one evening when the thrombotic infarct occurred. Ruth was transported to the nearby hospital, admitted to the intensive care unit, and later transferred to the acute care ward. It was three weeks since the stroke.

Years ago, the aphasiologist and the neuropsychologist agreed about the limitation of standardized aphasia and motor speech tests. They were aware that there are many schools of thought about aphasia and related disorders. They often quoted Henry Head's statement, made in the early 1900s, that aphasia is a "chaos" of classification systems. The aphasiologist and neuropsychologist decided that when discussing this patient, it would be best operationally to describe the symptoms. However, both agreed that Ruth displayed what most clinicians would call "Broca's aphasia with a predominance of apraxia of speech." Never ones to avoid a controversial subject, the aphasiologist and neuropsychologist began the brain localization debate with a factual review of the test results.

The aphasia evaluation showed that Ruth had mild initial difficulty following two and three-step commands and problems pointing to objects when named. There were also initial problems following complex written instructions. These initial receptive language difficulties resolved spontaneously within two weeks of the stroke. Expressive language remained impaired, with significant impairments describing common objects, completing sentences, imitating words and phrases, and with grammatical constructions. Ruth typically produced both literal and verbal paraphasias. As often happens with most expressive language disorders, Ruth's writing was typical of her verbal expression. She could not write sentences or names of objects, nor could she write to dictation. She could, however, copy printed words and simple geometric forms and sign her name. She also displayed moderate to severe dyscalculia.

The motor speech production testing showed moderate to severe apraxia of speech. Imitative production of vowels, continuants, plosives/affricates, and diphthongs were abnormal or nonfunctional. Longer, more complex motor speech programming, including one, two, and three syllable words, was also impaired. She displayed no success on multiple-word repetitions and phrase production. Ruth was aware of her errors most of the time, but was rarely self-corrective. Struggle was present on purposeful motor speech attempts. There were no indications of dysarthria.

Both the aphasiologist and the neuropsychologist agreed that crossed aphasia is the result of damage in the right hemisphere of the brain of a person who is definitively right-handed. The final agreement they reached that Saturday morning was that Ruth clearly met the criteria for diagnosis of crossed aphasia in a dextral, a rare aphasia occurring in fewer than 5 of every 100 cases.

The aphasiologist opined that Ruth was a fine example of the futility of localizing language to any particular part of the brain. He noted that localizationalists have spent, and continue to spend, time and energy, usually supported by large federal grants, to localize this, that, or another function to particular areas of the brain in all persons. He acknowledged that certain motor and sensory functions can be attributed to specific areas of the brain, but language is far too complex to be localized. He repeated that Ruth's aphasia was an example of the futility of efforts at localization. He reminded the neuropsychologist that Ruth's language functions are not confined to the typical Broca's or Wernicke's areas of the left hemisphere, but in her right brain, and he admonished his friend for being so short-sighted about these things.

The neuropsychologist praised his friend for accepting the proven localization of motor and sensory functions in the human brain. He reminded the aphasiologist that once he acknowledged that language can be localized to the brain, he has taken the first step to becoming a localizationalist. And as far as crossed aphasia is concerned, the qualification can easily be made that this type of aphasia can be localized to an infarction of the precentral gyrus in the right hemisphere of some right-handed persons. He observed that human neurology is complex and exploration of it should not be abandoned simply because of its complexity.

The aphasiologist acknowledged the complexity of human neurology and observed that the issue being debated involved language, arguably the most complex human neurological function. He criticized his friend for having a narrow definition of language—limiting it to labeling objects, events, and ideas. He suggested that thoughtful neuropsychogists should know language and thought are fundamentally intertwined in adult information processing. No better example of thought facilitating language and language facilitating thought could be found than Ruth's aphasia. While her nonverbal cognitive functions were relatively intact, her expressive language, including motor speech programming, was significantly impaired. Again, he reminded the neuropsychologist that Ruth's lesion was in her right hemisphere and about as far from Broca's area as one can get and remain in the brain.

The neuropsychologist praised the aphasiologist for his commitment to the obvious and observed that science has yet to understand thought and language. He told his friend it was presumptuous to believe language and thought facilitate each other given the limited scientific information currently available about either brain function. Cognitive psychology has made great advances in understanding how humans process information, but it has barely scratched the surface in knowing the complexities of cognition or language.

The aphasiologist and the neuropsychologist agreed to disagree about the merits of the localization movement, the nature of language and thought, and crossed aphasia in a dextral. They also agreed that continued scientific and philosophical exploration of these issues is essential to understanding language and cognition in humans and the myriad ways they can break down. They further agreed that regardless of the philosophical issues they debated that morning, their main concern was for Ruth and her rehabilitation. They turned their attention from lofty scientific and philosophical issues and began preparing treatment objectives and procedures for Ruth Lamb.

I am not one to make a mountain out of a mole hill, nor am I the kind of person to whistle past a graveyard, but I swear, they are out to get me. I put another smidgen of yellow scrambled egg on my tongue, press it to the roof of my mouth, and again challenge my taste buds to detect the powdery poison. There it is again. I can barely taste it, but something is definitely awry. Perhaps, it will be more discernible if I clean my palate with a gulp of water. I swish the water around in my mouth before testing the next deadly morsel. Again, a faint bitterness, just a hint of almond, but there it is. Have they sprinkled it on the eggs disguised as paprika? What did they think . . . I wouldn't notice? They are out to get me; it is not just in my mind. There is no question about it. Carefully, so as not to let them know I know, I bring a cloth napkin to my lips, and surreptitiously spit the deadly mouthful into it. So far, no one is the wiser. The waitress asks if all is well. I nod politely. It is better to say nothing. I hear the clack, clack, clack of the tracks as the train winds onward along the pacific coast, and I feel more helpless than ever. Soon, I hope, I will be in the safety of my small apartment just off Telegraph Avenue.

The train banks right as it rounds a costal peninsula and I must balance myself. Amazingly, the water glass and coffee cup manage to hold their contents with nary a drop spilled. Again, the waitress attends to me, commenting about the swaying ride and my abilities to manage it. I give her a gracious nod and pick at the rest of the breakfast, careful to avoid the eggs. I wonder if she is part of the plot to poison me. Nothing about her appearance or manner suggests she is a co-conspirator. Her doting ways, obvious attempts for maximum gratuity, are endearing, and I find myself strangely attracted to her. Her waitress badge identifies her as "Sharona," and she spends an inordinate amount of time with me, always smiling and upbeat. She is not drop-dead gorgeous, but attractive nonetheless. Her hair is cropped close to her scalp, accentuating dark eyes and even darker skin. Her waitress uniform unsuccessfully tries to hide her figure and I suspect no uniform or even a heavy tarp could do so. There is a vibrant body trying to spring from the cheap fabric, and for a few minutes, I fantasize about her sensual ways. I am so lonely, and it has been so long since I have had the warm embrace of a woman.

Chapter 2

Sunrise in San Francisco is a treat for the senses. Jack Sunday (his radio moniker) tightly ties his expensive running shoes and prepares to meet the morning sun, fog, rolling hills, and salt air of the City by the Bay. At six foot, Jack has that lean runner's look, and is one of the few men in his mid-40s who can wear spandex running shorts and not make pedestrians gag. His hair grayed early, much like his father's, but he keeps it short and never succumbs to the male ponytail sported by so many in show business. After two large gulps of water, two vitamins, and two full minutes of stretching, Jack Sunday trots down the long staircase to the street below. After a few more stretches, he begins the ritualized jog. At four in the morning there is no car competition, and Jack easily runs up Lombard Street smelling the roses and lilac bushes bordering the sharp curves of this famous San Francisco landmark. From Lombard Street, Jack lopes down the steep hill to the jogging trail winding along the shore to Fisherman's Wharf amid the pungent scent of fish and the early-morning shouts of vendors preparing for another day of tourists and townspeople. In the distance, a ship's low-pitched groan announces its arrival at this busy deep-water port. As the sun burns the remaining fog from the ocean, Alcatraz, in all its criminal glory, presents itself in the bay. At the ocean's edge, to the sounds of seals arguing over mackerel, Jack turns and begins to retrace his morning exercise tramp. He heads to the ancient, narrow four-story home where he and his wife Allyson have lived for nearly two decades. As the morning drive jock on KSSN, Jack's six figure income and generous stock options have made him one of the revered few, a homeowner in San Francisco. Jack knows he is blessed and, at least so far, life's journey has been an easy jog.

The return leg of the jog allows Jack to lose himself in thoughtful anticipation of the motorcycle road trip he and Allyson are to take. The two BMW cycles cost a pretty penny but are worth it. Twelve hundred cubic centimeters of German engineering power the bikes. The sleek two-wheelers are six-speed, counterbalanced, dream-machines with no pesky chains to tighten with Zen, or any other type, of motorcycle maintenance. Their seats and handgrips are heated, and global positioning satellites prevent the riders from losing their bearings. Jack and Allyson's red helmets, at nearly three hundred dollars, are state-of-the-art head protection. Black leather jackets, jackboots, and trousers provide further comfort and safety from rain, cold, and hard pavement should their bodies hit the highway at eighty miles-per-hour. No expense has been spared for the great motorcycle adventure through Yellowstone National Park. The final leg of Jack's jog is nearly vertical, and he is running late for work. He peeks through the garage window at the motorcycle marvels, and the freedom and adventure they are to bring. Still too early for Allyson, Jack showers, dresses, and leaves for downtown San Francisco and the early morning drive show. Dianne is already at the microphone when he arrives, the "on air" light flashes, and one hundred thousand watts of frequency-modulated power announce the "Jack and Dianne Show" to early morning San Franciscans. Nearly sixty percent of the market listens to the easy banter and light-hearted commentary intermixed with current and classic tunes for the city built on rock-and-roll.

Allyson is a slow-riser. While Jack is wide awake and ready for the world within ten minutes of his eyes opening, she needs two cups of strong coffee, the Chronicle, and at least an hour to fully regain her senses. After twenty-two years of marriage, it still irritates her that Jack is such a robust early-riser. And don't get Allyson started on joggers. She has and will continue to think of them as mentally ill, stricken with a disease that forces them to engage in sickening self-abuse for all to see. Early morning joggers are the worst of the ilk: disgusting creatures insanely pounding the pavement at daybreak when they should be sanely sleeping in the warm comfort of a bed. Jack learned long ago not to awaken Allyson, and to keep his early-morning, self-abusing ritual to himself. Once, early in their marriage, he woke her with an exercise invitation. Fortunately, with a lot of work, the marriage survived and she eventually forgave him.

The producers, advertisers, and sound engineers of the *Jack and Dianne Show* would prefer the stars never vacation, get sick, or in any way falter from the four hours of prime time radio programming. For years, the program has been a cash cow pushing KSSN to the top of the revenue charts. Advertising account executives demand, and get, obscene amounts of dollars from grateful businesses in the greater San Francisco area, and there is a waiting list of new advertisers vying for the precious radio time. Jack and Dianne have become as much a part of the San Francisco culture as the bridge, tower, and wharf of this sophisticated city. Dianne plays the sane, straight woman to the often outrageous Jack and his confusing but endearing views on life in the Bay Area. Besides his eccentric life views, Jack's unique semantics and his confused, but seemingly logical word usage delight audiences. Today in the studio, Dianne interviews two physicians from the city's professional football team, and Jack introduces them as a "paradox." Each show is punctuated with the apparently unrehearsed, unusual semantics that have become a hallmark of the *Jack and Dianne Show*. This summer, for the first time in several years, Jack and Dianne will take two weeks of needed vacation time, and KSSN will run the best segments, interviews, and commentaries in their place. At the conclusion of the show, Jack returns home and greets Allyson as she packs tents, sleeping bags, and camping supplies. Tomorrow morning, they will begin their great adventure.

The next morning, Jack opens his eyes, checks the clock, and sees that he has slept in. Last night, he and Allyson agreed he would jog as usual, awaken her at 7:00 a.m., and then they would begin their great adventure. ETD from the streets of San Francisco would be 8:00 a.m. Well, so much for precise planning. Jack thinks perhaps it is good to start the adventure flexibly, and for an instant, considers that an amorous morning romp with his wife would also be a fitting start to the vacation. He discards the thought as quickly as it was formed when he plays out in his mind her likely response to his suggestion of an early morning delight. In the past, Allyson has, for lack of a better word, discouraged

Jack from early morning sexual advances. Allyson's libido is also not an early riser and apparently, only a sex-crazed insane person would even suggest such a thing.

At eleven that morning, Jack and Allyson start their motorcycles, slowly coast down the driveway, cut through the downtown traffic, cross the Golden Gate Bridge, and spend the day cruising the wine country of northern California. That evening, they decide to spend the night in a cozy bed and breakfast rather than pitch a tent and rough it. After an early dinner, they tour a winery run by a brotherhood of monks and sample red, white, blush, and sparkling wines in a quaint wine cellar. Before going to bed, Jack replaces a burnt signal light bulb in his motorcycle, and as he crawls into bed, reports to Allyson that it was a necessary prefix to tomorrow's ride.

Day two of the great adventure begins at 10:00 a.m.—for Allyson, the crack of dawn. After a leisurely breakfast, Jack and Allyson carefully strap their overnight duffels to the backrests and tighten their tent and sleeping bags to the chrome storage racks of their motorcycles. They simultaneously start the engines, punch the foot shifters into first gear, ease the hand-held clutches, and follow a winding road to the interstate highway that will take them to Salt Lake City. At the freeway entrance, the adventurers open their throttles and smoothly hit the six gears until they speed through traffic like bright red bolts of light. The only custom work done to the motorcycles were handlebar extensions, back rests, and additional foot pedals placed high on the frame allowing the riders to lie back while the crotch rockets, as Jack calls them, speed toward Utah. They make good time, and by late evening, Jack and Allyson enter the large Mormon settlement and find a motel room. Again, they will forgo roughing it, and spend a comfortable night between bed sheets in an air-conditioned room. Like the early Mormon pioneers, they saddle up a little past daybreak (in Allyson hours, 9:30 a.m.), and head toward the Idaho state line. Traffic is light, the weather warm and sunny, and by nightfall, they enter West Yellowstone, Montana. They stay the night in a rustic log cabin and approach the west entrance of the park the next morning. As planned, they will spend four days and three nights touring the nation's oldest and grandest national park.

Chapter 3

This job was simply to be a temporary gig. No way was being a hospital orderly a lifelong career choice for Clarence. He simply wanted to earn enough money to pay for the new speakers, catch up on his rent, and buy some used stage lights. Clarence kept reminding himself that it really is all about the music, and his fledgling band was starting to show signs of taking off. At long last, the band was doing fewer airport motel lounges and frat parties, and more dances, even if some were only at high schools. The latest invitation to be an opening act at the university concert was the first real sign that his unique retro rhythm and soul blues was more than yet another garage band. Good things were beginning to happen, and for twenty-five year old Clarence, it was about time. He would continue to suffer the indignities of bedpans, unruly patients, and meal trays for the needed money because it really is about the music. This temporary hospital gig was now three years old. Clarence crushes the cigarette into the gravel, winks at Connie, and leaves the designated smoking area and the rest of the nicotine-crazed outcasts shivering in the cold. It is time to transport a patient to radiology.

Connie carefully times her smoking breaks to spend them with Clarence. The eighteen-year-old doesn't like the smoking habit, really only lights up at work, and only when it means time with Clarence and smokers' small talk. Connie can take or leave the cigarettes, but not Clarence, for she is hopelessly mesmerized by the budding musician. To others, Clarence is just another orderly in a dead-end job, but Connie sees through all of that. Clarence is going to make it, and if Connie has her way, he will make it with her. She returns his wink with a smile; just enough to acknowledge him, but not so much as to show her burning desire to explore exciting possibilities. After Clarence is out of sight, Connie discards the partially smoked cigarette and returns to the fourth floor nurses' station where she is the ward clerk.

Clarence enjoys transporting patients from one part of this huge medical campus to another. He especially likes moving patients from the rehabilitation center to the radiology department because they are at the extreme ends of the medical complex. When he arrives on the fourth floor, he is told the patient is in the dining room. Clarence enters the busy dining room to a blast of curious odors. He detects the pleasant smells of coffee, toast, and possibly bacon, as well as the not-so-pleasant odor of sick and hurt people poorly camouflaged by acrid disinfectant. The patient is a head injury and one of the more bizarre ones. Rumor has it that he is hypersexual, and hits on every female he sees. Clarence politely waits for the nurses' aide and some kind of therapist to finish their business with him. They are cleaning him and his wheelchair after a messy bout with food nearly toppling to the floor. A restraint vest tightly secures him to his wheelchair and his arms are tied to the armrests. Last week during a smoking break, Connie told Clarence of this patient's right hook and the bloodied nose of the nurse who was trying to dress him. The patient, R414 as he is known in medical records, has post-traumatic psychosis and is a level-two danger to him self and the staff.

Clarence approaches R414 as the therapist leaves. She is obviously unnerved by the last round of propositions, sexual innuendo, and suggestive tongue movements that would make KISS envious. Leaning down to unlock the wheelchair, Clarence is suddenly the object of a restrained kick to the head. Narrowly missing the assault, Clarence takes the handles of the wheelchair and begins transporting R414 to radiology. The patient curses several times in the dining room and questions Clarence's parentage. At the nurses' station, Clarence jokingly asks Connie if using duct tape on R414 mouth would be inappropriate. She suggests it would be frowned upon by the hospital administration, but is nonetheless a great idea. Clarence wheels the chair to the elevator knowing this transport is likely to be an eventful one. Fortunately, they are alone in the elevator and it is a straight shot to the ground floor. R414 is finally quiet and seems to enjoy the ride. They are accompanied by an elevator rendition of "Light My Fire," apparently conducted by the Boston Pops. Clarence thinks the tune is enough to make Jim Morrison do a 360 in his Parisian grave, and to cause R414 to break from his restraints. "What next?" Clarence asks the patient. "Frank Sinatra does Pink Floyd's 'We . . . don't . . . need . . . no . . . education, HEY!, leave . . . us . . . kids . . . alone, HEY!'"

Clarence takes music seriously and R414 concurs by uttering the f-word. At last they agree on something, and Clarence senses something likable about R414.

Chapter 4

The lines are long at the West Entrance to Yellowstone National Park. Allyson crawls a car-length at a time in her line, and Jack does the same in a separate one. At the same time, they both reach the rangers taking money, passing out fliers and maps, and warning the tourists, especially those on motorcycles, to watch out for bears. Allyson and Jack drive about three hundred yards beyond the entrance gate and review the maps. They decide to motor first to Mammoth Hot Springs, past Tower Fall (yes, "Fall" not "Falls"), over the highest mountain in the park, and then to Canyon Village. From Canyon Village, they will divert to Old Faithful. How could they tour Yellowstone and not see this famous geyser? From Old Faithful, they will see Fishing Bridge and the large, breathtaking, pine-bordered Yellowstone Lake. Then, they will exit the park and drive the short distance to Jackson Hole, Wyoming, and home to San Francisco. The scent of pine trees, fresh air, and excitement is in the air. As they cruise in third gear through the pine-shadowed road, they parallel Madison River snaking from higher elevation to the lowlands. On the river they see wild swans, ducks, and geese, and to their right is a large expanse of grass and clover with at least twenty buffalo grazing on it. (Apparently, in Yellowstone, they are called bison; "You say tomato, I say buffalo," thinks Jack.) Jack takes in the scenery and mutters: "Yellowstone, Allyson, and the BMWs; it just doesn't get any better than this."

At Madison Junction and the first stop sign, they see a rustic marker suggesting a short detour along Fire Hole Drive. They turn onto the very small paved road, travel through the deep canyon, and reach high cliffs where daring people dive nearly 50 feet into the warm, spring-fed river. Jack and Allyson decide not to attempt the derring-do, cruise the remaining drive, and return to Madison Junction. Ten minutes later, they are hit by a blast of sulfur odor emanating from several bubbling hot pots. They park their motorcycles in the lot and walk the wooden-plank path through them. Several teenagers, workers at the park's trinket shops and cafes, discuss "hot pottin." Apparently, late at night the locals sneak naked into the lukewarm ones and enjoy their youth and nature spas. Returning to their bikes, Allyson comments that it is a little disconcerting knowing that they are touring a live volcano with so much heat and energy just below the surface.

Riding parallel, Jack and Allyson cruise through the magnificent scenery. Yellowstone is a wonderful motorcycle tour with eagles soaring above them, streams and waterfalls, moose, elk, deer, antelope, mountain sheep, and buffalo. About thirty miles into the park, they encounter their first "bear jam." There has been a sighting of this famous Yellowstone icon, and the cars are stopped in the middle of the road to see it. The traffic is backed for nearly a mile, and there is no room for cars to pass. Motorcycles, however, have special freedom. Allyson and Jack cruise carefully between the rows of cars and are soon at the bear sighting. Just to the side of the road, in a grove of young lodge pole pine trees, are a large brown bear and her cub. Tourists surround them snapping pictures, pointing, and exclaiming how privileged they are to be witnessing such an event. They appear oblivious to the danger should they get between the mother bear and her cub. Jack and Allyson remain on their motorcycles in case a quick exit is required. Soon, they are at Mammoth, the administrative center of the park, and home of a colorful volcanic mountain. They park their bikes at one of the log-constructed cafes and enjoy an expensive lunch. Then, they start their motorcycles with one easy press of a starter button and prepare to climb to the high country of Yellowstone. First, though, they must cross a narrow bridge over a deep canyon. It is on this bridge that Jack will have his brush with death.

The metal bridge is at least one thousand feet above a small creek flowing through a steep-walled canyon. From one side to the other, it is about the length of two football fields. It is much narrower than the road leading to and from it, and is barely wide enough for two cars. Obviously built before modern automobiles, the metal span could easily accommodate Model A and T Fords, but barely two Toyota Land Cruisers. Two iron rails, about four feet high, border the narrow bridge. Jack and Allyson ride single file and speed toward the death trap.

Sagebrush bordering the side of the road leading to the bridge dances in the light wind. Jack enters the bridge first, and fortunately, both he and Allyson are the only vehicles on it. About midpoint, a gust of wind blows through the canyon, and the BMW is hit with forty miles-per-hour of invisible force. Jack's motorcycle is blown into the oncoming lane, and he leans the bike nearly on its side to avoid the steel barrier. As Jack avoids a skid, it dawns upon him, in perfect clarity, how the barrier is just high enough to block the motorcycle from falling hundreds of feet to the creek below, but not high enough to prevent him from flying unimpeded into the great expanse and eternity. During this slow motion epiphany, Jack realizes just how close he is to death, for he feels no fear, no anxiety. In a matter-of-fact assessment of the situation, he sees how his life will end and the events that have led up to this point in time. As he prepares to lay the bike on its side, the wind stops just as fast as it began. He is able to right the motorcycle, return to his lane, and avoid disaster. Allyson, seeing Jack's plight, brakes with both the handlebar and foot brakes, and successfully avoids a similar crisis. They re-group on the other side. Jack's hands are shaking, his face is pale, and for the first time in his life, he knows his mortality.

Chapter 5

Maybe I should try to sleep what with the soothing sound of the train tracks. The clack, clack, clack monotony, and the relentless swaying of the train may let me relax, put down my defenses just for a few hours, and get some needed shuteye. Just as I standup, there is a jolt to the train's sway, and I nearly topple to the floor. Righting myself, I accidently brush against the waitress. Her role, if any, in the plot to kill me is unknown, but I must suspect everyone. I quickly check her hands for a shiv or other sharp object, and finding none, I politely offer a "Thank you" for her assistance. A porter leads the way past other diners and through the whooshing pneumatic sliding doors.

I know of the terrorists' plot, and I know they know I know. To the religious radicals, San Francisco is the belly of the beast. If the United States is the great Satan, then San Francisco must represent all that is evil, even more so than the partially destroyed New York. If the terrorists have their way, the destruction of my beloved city will happen soon. Tens of thousands of San Franciscans, including everyone I love, will lose their lives to a bunch of stone-age, cave-dwelling zealots. I must impart the method and means of their madness to the powers-that-be. The train ends its run in Oakland, and I will have only a few minutes to alert them. It will be a race against time, and if I lose, thousands will die an agonizing, slow death at the hands of these lowlife monsters. But I am exhausted, and as I have been taught, with fatigue comes mistakes. I covertly scan my surroundings, ever alert to the slightest irregularity, suspicious of everyone and everything. There is too much at stake to let my guard down even for a moment, for if I fail, all is lost.

Reaching my sleeping compartment, I carefully lock the door and draw the heavy industrial curtain. This small compartment is a steel uterus protecting me from the outside and giving me temporary reprieve from danger. The clack, clack, clack heartbeat further gives me a sense of security as I lie on the small bed. I can barely hear the other passengers talking, laughing, and moving from dining car to their first-class accommodations. I know the terrorists are on the train, plotting and planning my demise and the death of San Francisco. This time, airplanes will not be crashing into defenseless buildings: it will be a dirty bomb. While the homeland defense team mindlessly fights the last war, carefully removing box knives and innocent Arabs from passenger airplanes, the terrorists have moved on. They will use microbes to cleanse more infidels from their heaven-on-earth psychotic glory.

To me, what is most ironic about the terrorists' hatred is that San Francisco is the most "live and let live" city in the United States. San Franciscans are tolerant of others and repress no one. Yet these crazed lunatics will kill thousands of them, senselessly, brutally, and with malicious forethought, all in the name of their God. In their sick minds, nonbelievers must believe, and all heathen heretics must die. I have never been a religious man and it is difficult for me to fathom this myopic mentality, and the mindless maniacs who are driven by it. Well, they've met their match with me and I'll notify the authorities and as many citizens as possible. They made a big mistake discussing the plot in Arabic, not knowing that I too speak the ancient language. They made a bigger mistake not knowing that sound travels very well from compartment to compartment through the air conditioning. Finally, I drift into the sanctuary of a half-sleep to the clack, clack, clack of the train. My sleep is disturbed by random, unconnected dreams of being moved through a narrow passage to a dimly lit interrogation room, where a seductive female terrorist futilely tries to extract information. In my fragmented dreams, they must break me. They must discover what I know, when I learned it, and who I have told. Oh, they are good at interrogation, and even in my dreams, I respect the tenacity of the despicable sons-of-bitches.

Chapter 6

"R414 seems placid enough," thinks Clarence, "Maybe this will be an uneventful transport after all." On the bottom floor of the rehabilitation unit, Clarence wheels R414 through the wide hall past several staff and an elderly couple with a flower bouquet in hand, apparently on their way to visit a relative. The patient watches the people with a quiet intensity, his hands forcefully grasping the armrests of the wheelchair. Clarence sees the white knuckles and sweat beads forming on R414's forehead, and asks him if all is well. He kneels down in front of the patient, and is momentarily startled by the madman look on the distraught patient's face. He sees sheer terror in the piercing eyes, and suddenly is spat upon.

"You bastard. Bastard, bastard, bastard. I'll kill you," slurs R414. His hands and feet test the strength of the restraints, jerking and pulling in a desperate attempt to break free.

"Easy does it, partner," Clarence replies in his most low-pitched, soothing voice. "We're going to get an X-ray."

Again, R414 spouts profanity like a machine gun, each disgusting rapid-fire epitaph loud enough for all to hear. After a brief pause, the staff members continue on their way and the elderly couple, obviously startled, stares silently at them. Clarence reassures them all is well, and that the patient is just agitated. Again, R414 pulls, jerks, and struggles at the restraints. For a moment, Clarence is afraid they will break and release the psycho; tomorrow's newspaper will show pictures of the carnage and the headline will read: "R and B Musician Killed in Hospital Assault."

Apparently, one of the passing staff members told Connie of the disturbance and she and an RN arrive just in time to see R414 make one final attempt to break free from the restraints. The nurse, sedative in hand, prepares to give the shot to the patient. Then, just as rapidly as it started, R414 calms down, offers a slanted smile, and says, "I'm done. There's no need for that."

He turns his head to Connie and says, "My, but that is an attractive color for you." Although garbled, the compliment seems genuine and she graciously accepts it. The RN postpones the needle, and Clarence, now with the RN and Connie as backup, continues with the transport of the patient.

At this hospital complex, there is a glass-enclosed walkway spanning a busy city street. With the RN and Connie following, they begin the trek through the arching tower. Clarence casually pushes R414 through the glass tunnel that will eventually take them to the radiology section. Several scrub nurses and a respiratory therapist approach from the other side of the walkway, and as they pass, R414 suddenly frees his left arm from the restraint and reaches for them. One of the scrub nurses is a small woman in her early 20s. She is slim with orange-red, curly hair, and is wearing granny glasses that give her an attractive librarian facade. She is also too slow to avoid his lunge. R414 tears at her blue surgical uniform, grasps her by the wrist, and pulls the frightened woman down to him.

"Jan, Paul, So In," he whispers through gritted teeth.

His barely intelligible words register no meaning with the distraught nurse, and she replies, "Let me alone."

Clarence, Connie, and the RN quickly restrain R414, pry his fingers from her wrist, and apologize profusely for the assault. "Head injury," Connie explains, and the two words satisfactorily sum the incident to the scrub nurse. She and R414's eyes meet for one last nonverbal exchange. His expression is one of fear and desperation. Graciously accepting the apology, the scrub nurse rearranges her uniform, and continues on her way, no worse for wear. Again, R414 is firmly secured to his wheelchair, and they continue with more care so the incident will not be repeated.

The remainder of the odyssey is completed with no more assaults, and finally they reach the radiology department. Connie and the RN bid Clarence and R414 adieu and leave. Clarence checks in with the department secretary, and after a brief wait, wheels R414 into the examination room. The room is dimly lit, and only dark images of high-tech instruments can be seen. In the corner is a hospital bed with the head raised to a partially upright position. A television monitor secured by a metal frame hangs from the ceiling, and there is a futuristic, black, conical X-ray device for directing streams of invisible atomic particles into patients. Clarence hears a low-pitched hum as he waits with R414 for the radiology personnel to begin the diagnostic. The patient starts to show signs of agitation, and Clarence wonders how this procedure will end.

After a long wait, providing ample time for R414's paranoid thoughts to fester, a radiologist and his assistant enter the room. A therapist, the one so obviously unnerved by R414's round of propositions, sexual innuendo, and suggestive tongue movements, enters the room and briefly discusses how they will position the patient. They don heavy, lead-lined aprons to protect themselves from radiation, and Clarence is told to unstrap R414 from his chair. Clarence suggests this is not a good idea and recounts the walkway incident. He is told that to complete the test, R414 must be placed on the examination bed, and Clarence does what he is told.

"We are going to put you on the bed for the X-ray test," he informs R414. The restraints are removed, and R414 calmly lies on the bed and permits new restraints to be used. Clarence is surprised at how amenable R414 is to the procedure. The bed is adjusted to an upright position, and the long conical tube is placed to the patient's head and neck. On the monitor, his blurry skeleton can be seen. R414 shows no anger or fear, and the lights dim several times as the first X-rays are taken. Then, the therapist holds a white liquid in a paper cup to the patient's mouth and asks him to drink it. Again, R414 calmly consents and takes several swallows of the chalky substance. On the monitor, the liquid enters his skeletal mouth and is swallowed. He coughs several times, but shows no distress at the procedure. Finally, everyone removes their lead aprons, R414 is placed in his chair, and they return to rehabilitation center without incident. Clarence is surprised at how easily the test was conducted, and praises R414 for a job well done.

Chapter 7

Certainly, Jack has always known he is mortal and eventually he will die. The very definition of mortal means, "destined to die." Everyone knows at an early age that their days are numbered. After regrouping and collecting themselves on the safe side of the bridge, this time with Allyson in the lead, Jack hits second gear and understands that until today, at least for him, death was a premise. His loss of life was to be some vague ending far into the future. Third gear brings another realization to Jack: feeling one's mortality and knowing it are two different perceptions. Intellectualizing the fact that all living things end and feeling fear, despair, and confusion at one's own not-so-distant certain demise are at the extremes of human perception. Jack also comprehends that besides death, there are many other types of loss, and the bridge has caused a loss of his innocence. Shifting into fourth gear, he knows the bridge has forever changed his life, and he no longer has the youthful privilege of perceiving his death as an abstraction.

For the BMW, cruising speed through the park is fifth gear, keeping the RPMs nearly at an idle and allowing quiet for easy reflection. Jack leans against the backrest and lifts his feet into position on the frame, and has his final realization: there really was a death on Mammoth Bridge today. Never-ending Jack died, and so too did his sense of invincibility. Death now rides with Jack on the BMW through the rolling hills, the small scrub pines, and the narrow road leading to Roosevelt Lodge (where they have reservations for a real wild-west horseback ride and camping trip). They gear down to slow their descent into the valley as Roosevelt lodge, the riding stables, and circled wagons appear to their right. They pull into the large gravel parking lot, only this time Jack slows to first gear, trailing far behind Allyson. Gravel can be dangerous for two-wheelers, especially when trying to stop using the front brake. Jack takes no unnecessary chances, what with his new, dark passenger.

An hour later, Allyson and Jack saddle-up under the careful supervision of the trail boss and ride gentle horses single-file into the backwoods of Yellowstone. There are twelve other tourists, "dudes," and a canvas-covered chuck wagon follows the procession. Waterfalls, babbling brooks, and hordes of wild park animals highlight the three-mile ride. They make camp; eat steak, beans, and biscuits; sing "Camp Town Ladies;" and sleep under the vast expanse of the western sky. That night as Jack lies under millions of sparkling stars, he ponders the passage of time, the meaning of it all, and the tune "Dust in the Wind." As usual, he awakens early and sits alone by the glowing coals of the campfire, contemplating God and the infinite as the sun peeks over the mountainous Yellowstone sky.

That morning, Jack and Allyson are first in line on the return horse procession to Roosevelt Lodge. Jack comments to the trail boss that some trailers are having a difficult time keeping up. The trail boss, after grappling with the semantics of his statement, slows the lead horses, and soon all the dudes are in a compact line. By noon, Allyson and Jack straddle their motorcycles, climbing higher into the mountains of Yellowstone. They stop briefly at Tower Fall to witness the grand spectacle. From Tower Fall, they ascend even higher to a road sign showing an elevation of more than 10,000 feet above sea level. They contemplate the reality that they are nearly two miles closer to the sun than at their four-story home in San Francisco.

Descending into Canyon Village, they encounter their second bear jam. A brown bear is standing on two feet, feasting on Twinkies and sandwiches offered through small cracks in car windows. Apparently, tourists disregard the admonition, "Do Not Feed the Bears." At one car, a woman has smeared peanut butter on her child's arm and is busily taking pictures of the bear licking it from the youngster. Seeing the stupid spectacle, Jack ponders how sacred life is and how mortals seem to take it for granted. Since the bridge, Jack knows that life is as fragile as a dream, and he will never again take it for granted. Hendrix's "Are You Experienced?" echoes in his head.

Canyon Village is a bustling tourist center and a major Yellowstone crossroad. There is a large log-constructed hotel, a gas station, trinket shops, cafes, and two grocery stores. At the junction, Jack and Allyson stop and read the detailed wooden road sign with white lettering listing alternatives to their journey. Turning right at the junction will return them to the West Entrance of the park, Montana and Idaho, and the small town of West Yellowstone. Turning left apparently will take them to the namesake of the tourist center and the Grand Canyon of the Yellowstone. The brochure shows it to be a smaller facsimile of the Arizona mile-deep tribute to erosion and evolution. Continuing straight ahead will take them to Fishing Bridge, Lake Village, and eventually the Grand Tetons and Jackson Hole, Wyoming. Adhering to their carefully planned itinerary, Allyson and Jack take the 30-mile side trip to Old Faithful and the heart of Yellowstone's volcanic energy.

As he rides parallel though the forest-lined, narrow road, Jack watches Allyson through the corners of his eyes and marvels at her mettle and tenacity as she shifts through the BMW's six gears. Having spent more than two decades with her, he now looks at her with different eyes since Mammoth Bridge and the boarding of his new shadowy passenger. He has the sad realization that she and all the other tourists he has met on life's journey are strangers at heart. He is close to Allyson physically and mentally. The intimacies they have shared certainly bridged their consciousness, and perhaps that is the real powerful driving force behind the human need for them. Physically, mentally, and emotionally they have shared the high and low roads of life's pilgrimage thus far. But they really have not known each other's consciousness and awareness; they have only occasionally connected.

Her hair flutters behind her helmet as she speeds through the bright, sunny Yellowstone day. With Jack, she has been independent yet intimate, aloof and familiar, distant and chummy. But who is Allyson? What thoughts reside behind those ethereal jet-black eyes? What is she saying to herself as she nods and smiles at him nearly hidden in that expensive red helmet? Has Allyson also made room for a dark passenger on her pilgrimage? When did he board? For a brief moment, Jack wonders if Allyson might just be another mindless prop in this elaborate life hoax. Perhaps, Jack fears, Allyson has no thoughts. Perchance Jack rides solo. That damnable Mammoth Bridge has shaken Jack's sense of reality.

So far, Yellowstone National Park has lived up to its hype. It is a splendid vacation site, albeit one with danger and unwanted riders. To some, fools who smear peanut butter on a child's arm as a photo opportunity, the park is Disneyland on a larger scale. Notwithstanding stupid people, Yellowstone is not Nature Land in a commercial amusement park; it is primal nature at its best and at its worst. Life, death, and survival play out every day in this vast untouched wilderness just beyond the highways and trails. Jack leans into a tight curve, and approaches the Village of Old Faithful. He thinks about nature, fairness, and brutality. Predator wolves, coyotes, and cougars tear flesh from elk, rabbits, and deer. Not from the fastest and fittest, but from the weak, old, and newborns. Life seems so unjust and unfair, and Yellowstone captures it in all its brutal glory. For Jack, death and dying are everywhere and there is no escaping it.

Then, Jack and Allyson approach an anachronism, something clearly out of place in this grand spectacle. To get to Old Faithful Geyser, they must take a freeway clover leaf. Yes, a cloverleaf. Out of the blue on this picturesque, narrow highway, there appears a Los Angeles cloverleaf! The park has been carefully, almost religiously, kept and maintained to minimize the human element, and yet some rocket surgeon has placed a freeway cloverleaf in plain view of grazing moose, hawks stalking prey, and bubbling mud pots. Four lanes, an underpass, and green freeway signs direct Jack and Allyson to Old Faithful. What major brain fart created this tribute to so-called civilization? What next, fast food joints, billboards, graffiti-splattered walls, and drive-through liquor stores lining the freeway to Old Faithful?

Parking their motorcycles in a large lot, Allyson and Jack walk the small, rock-lined trail to the viewing area and sit on large, fallen tree trunks carefully lined for witnessing the spectacle. Jack listens intently to a Rangerette as she waxes on and on about the workings of this geyser. The molten heat emanating from the earth's hellish core boils water until it no longer can contain the energy. Then Old Faithful blows its stack, sending torrents of water and steam high into the Yellowstone sky. Precisely on time, the ground vibrates and the geyser roars to life, again to the ever-present, incessant clicking of cameras. Jack wonders how many relatives and neighbors will be forced to sit through hours of photographic records of this and other vacation experiences. Long ago, Jack and Allyson decided not to be shutterbugs on life's journey. They agreed not to see life through a view finder while reading f-stops. They agreed not to miss the moment by trying to capture it. After Old Faithful is spent, Jack asks Allyson when again the molten id below the geyser will force another timely orgasm.

Chapter 8

I am jarred from my half-sleep by two male insurgents arguing in that disgusting Arabic tone over my plight. The third terrorist, Sharona, is the waitress from the dining car, still wearing her food-server uniform, still failing to hide her sensual curves, and still seductive with her Middle Eastern male-pleasuring ways. These terrorists are no dummies, for they know my weakness. They know of my loneliness and my passion for dark-eyed women. Sharona's alluring bouquet spellbinds me and I feel her body heat as she brushes against me. We share a spot of English-style tea, heavy on the cream, as she questions me about my knowledge of their plot. I pretend to speak only English and haphazardly answer her queries. Between sips of Earl Grey, I see in her eyes a need to be with me, to abandon the murderous plot, and to do the right thing. Perhaps, she is a double agent, planted among the axis of evil to derail their treachery. I sense she wants me to play along, and I will, at least long enough to reach San Francisco and alert the citizenry. Then, as suddenly as the interrogation began, I find myself alone again in the sleeping compartment, accompanied only by the clack, clack, clack of steel wheels on iron rails.

Chapter 9

Today, Connie resolves, she will make her interest in Clarence known. She matter-of-factly announces to no one in particular that today she will help transport R414, and considers topics she could broach as a bridge to the captivating musician. Should she confess to Clarence that she has faithfully attended his concerts, or would he mistake her R & B interest as stalking? During smoking breaks, should she request a light for her cigarette, and in a Greta Garbo seductive contrive, gently hold his hand during the light and pose a sensual pout? No, she thinks, far too obvious. After weighing several options, finally she resolves to use the antics of R414 as an icebreaker, certainly something interesting they share. R414 will be a bridge to their everlasting happiness.

Chapter 10

Jack and Allyson tour Old Faithful Village and shop several souvenir stores. On their return to San Francisco, as promised, they will give their friends and family curios, baubles, knickknacks, and bric-a-bracs attesting to their great adventure in the Yellowstone wilderness. Allyson finds sensible mementos of the trip. Jack, however, struggles for the perfect memorabilia for Dianne. What to buy? He considers wild-west hats, vests with pictures of bears, tomahawks with blue and green feathers glued to their handles, and pocket knives with pictures of geysers. The Korean-made cache of trinkets and toys are treasures for the hordes of children begging cash-strapped parents for keepsakes. But, what would suit Dianne? What would symbolize their friendship and capture the Yellowstone essence, but more importantly, show his thoughtfulness and sophistication? Since the boarding of his malignant companion at Mammoth Bridge, he has a newfound appreciation of Dianne's raillery, repartee, and radio ways. "Some people are so hard to buy for," he tells Allyson, as a perky teenager swipes her credit card and bags five impeccably appropriate gifts. Jack searches more isles and examines rubber Bowie knives, boxed rocks of different colors, and a book of magician tricks. Leather belts and white T-shirts with Yellowstone National Park printed on them, hiking shoes, and saltwater taffy confound Jack even further in his quest for the ideal gift. Finally, after an hour of approach-avoidance conflicts and Allyson's increasing impatience, Jack leaves the store with a small plastic replica of the Golden Gate Bridge for his comrade Dianne. Riding through the village, Jack looks in the bag at the bridge replica, shakes his head, and utters over the hum of the motorcycle: "Stupid, stupid, stupid. Some people are so hard to buy for."

Finding an available campsite at Old Faithful is challenging, but finally, after nearly an hour of searching, Allyson and Jack luck out. This campground, teeming with children noisily running from one campsite to another, is surrounded by and saturated with pine trees. Each campsite has a metal barbeque, a campfire pit lined by small rocks, and a smooth area to lie atop sleeping bags. They pitch their tent, unpack cooking supplies, and carefully lay out sleeping bags. As the sun sets over the top of the trees, they build a small campfire, brew coffee, chat, and watch gray smoke from the fire drift upward. After a dinner of cheeseburgers, Allyson reads a dime-store novel by the light of the flickering campfire. There is tranquility to the camp, but unexpectedly, Jack has a flood of melancholy. Later, as Allyson rests, tucked comfortably in tent and sleeping bag, Jack sits quietly alone feeding dead grass to the glowing coals. The grim reaper who boarded on Mammoth Bridge mockingly sits next to Jack on the smooth rock. He wonders about the meaning of it all and again is overwhelmed with loneliness. He wonders if all the philosophy courses he took in college have prepared him for this crisis.

For Jack, before Mammoth Bridge, existentialism was an intellectual exercise taught by depressive atheists like Jean-Paul Sartre and Søren Kierkegaard. Certainly, in college, the philosophy had a true ring to it and gave much needed accountability to the human condition. Too much evil has been done by religious extremists, the Devil, and soldiers just following orders. But existentialism, like Jack's inevitable demise, was simply an academic exercise with no real connection to his world. Now, as he sits alone (and lonely) at the Yellowstone campfire, he finds an appreciation of the limits of his reality. As he ponders the nature of human consciousness, a small chipmunk scampers to his foot and makes eye-contact, nonverbally begging for a scrap of food. Jack complies with a bread crumb, and it returns to its camp with nary a thanks. Jack fondles the miniature replica of the Golden Gate Bridge and wonders if the chipmunk knows it is a chipmunk, and if it ever ponders eternity and the great abyss. Does the small creature ever wonder what it is like to be a squirrel? Jack decides to keep the plastic bridge and to find another gift for Dianne.

Like millions of humans before him during times of spiritual crisis, Jack turns to religion for solace and protection. But that too is small comfort. Jack has never been one to personify the universe. At least from his perspective, Jack realizes that doctrine and dogma are as irrational as atheism. He understands that the despair he feels is one of not knowing, and atheists and believers alike are fooling themselves. Had Jack hurtled over Mammoth Bridge, flailing and screaming into eternity, he wonders if the answers to life mysteries would have been revealed before his body crashed to the rocks below, just before the spark of his awareness forever darkened. A tear slips down his left cheek as he bids final farewell to his invincibility, and begins the long road leading to acceptance of the unacceptable. Jack sits at the smoldering campfire more alone than he has ever been. He wonders if a lifetime of Prozac is an antidote to existential despair. He thinks it ironic that this emptiness began on a bridge. Later, as he slides into his sleeping bag, he realizes that he finally knows the meaning to the "Hotel California" lyrics.

Chapter 11

Clarence's pager signals another R414 transport. Connie at the nurses' station says R414 and three other patients are to be taken to "reality orientation," which Clarence gathers is some type of group therapy for head injured patients. When Clarence arrives at R414's room, the patient has been dressed and placed in his wheelchair. Clarence thinks R414 looks quite dapper in his casual attire, and surprisingly normal. He is wearing black slacks, argyle socks, loafers, and a dark blue sweater over a lighter blue turtleneck. The new growth of his hair is now manageable with a brush and hair gel. Apparently, restraints are no longer necessary, unless, as Clarence suspects, they are invisible, chemical ones. R414 appears docile, but as Clarence has found, appearances can be deceptive. Guardedly, Clarence greets R414, unlocks his wheel breaks, and begins the transport to the group therapy suite. Connie joins them in hall with chart in hand and will accompany them. At the elevator door, Clarence remarks that it is a fine morning, and R414 concurs with an intelligible, but slurred reply. In the elevator, they are crooned to by Frank Sinatra's declaration that he has traveled life's road "his way." R414 looks up and back at Clarence with a facial expression suggesting impending nausea. Clarence wonders aloud if the elevator industry will ever embrace rap, subjecting trapped riders to chamber music about "hoes" and "dissen." Connie laughs and R414 concurs. Clarence winks and smiles at the likeable patient, knowing they are both rock-and-roll purists.

When they reach the group therapy room, three other head injured patients are seated in a row facing a chalk board. They are a motley crew with shorn, scarred scalps, drooling, and stuporous expressions. Next to the chalkboard are pictures of hospitals, doctors, nurses, clocks, and a large-print calendar pinned to poster board. There are more therapists and aides than patients. When R414's wheels are locked in place, the session is called to order by a very serious middle-aged woman in a white uniform. She asks Clarence to remain during the session in case things get out of control.

Clarence and Connie stand at the rear of the large room. The therapist begins the first of what she promises will be many sessions to help the three men and one woman re-learn who they are, what happened to them, and other important aspects of life and living. They will re-learn family, friends, and pets. She goes on to explain that they must learn temporal events such as birthdays, holidays, and to appreciate the passage of time. Each patient will again know what they did for a living, where they lived, and many other facets about their life before the traumatic brain injury. According to the therapist, a rewarding time will be had by all. She then asks each patient for his or her name, and applauds when they are uttered correctly or nearly correctly. She then points to a picture of the hospital and asks, "What is this?"

R414 sits dutifully during the introduction and appears to be going along with the program. A teenage girl with a large, white head bandage sits next to him, and they briefly exchange glances. The other two head injured patients, both in their 20s, appear oblivious to the purpose of the meeting, but are watchful nonetheless. The therapist kneels down to eye-level with R414 and asks if he can describe the building in the picture. Clarence moves closer to them should R414 take a swing at her. In response to her question, R414 calmly says the picture is of a government building and mumbles something about "the fall of the tower." The therapist then asks the others in the group if R414 is correct. There is a general hum of agreement, and the therapist explains that it is indeed a building, but is a hospital where sick and injured people are helped, and there is no tower to fall. Then, one of the men begins crying, and the teenager covers her face with her hands. R414 utters a string of nonsensical statements ostensibly relating to the mistake the doctors have made. Apparently, there has been some major error in medical judgment by placing him with the rest of the group. Evidently, R414 is simply in the building to answer bureaucratic questions, and he is perfectly normal. At the conclusion of the garbled statements, R414 asks the therapist if she would kindly urge the crying man to "shut up." He turns his head to Clarence, rolls his eyes, clearly expressing that he has been cast into a group of psychos and will tolerate it no longer.

Clarence prepares himself for a disturbance should R414 attempt to escape from reality orientation. Then out of the blue, R414 breaks into song: "They're going to take me away, ha, ha, hee hee. They're going to lock me up, ha ha, hee, hee." Both Connie and Clarence recognize the silly tune from the early 60s, and laugh uncontrollably. The therapist gives Connie and Clarence a look of displeasure, and asks R414 to stop singing. Now both men are crying and the teenage girl is peeking at the cuckoo theater through her fingers. R414 responds to the therapist's request to stop singing by doing it louder: "They're going to take me away, ha ha, hee, hee. They're going to lock me up."

The first crying man is now shouting, "Looney tunes, looney tunes. Looney tunes, looney bin." The second crying man begins shouting obscenities through crying sobs.

The therapist asks Clarence to return R414 to his room, and as they leave reality orientation, the patient breaks into Steppenwolf's anthem to easy riders: "Born to be Wild." Clarence whispers to Connie that the first session of reality orientation did not go too well.

Chapter 12

Uncharacteristically, Allyson awakes before Jack, cooks bacon and eggs, and percolates coffee while he sleeps soundly in the tent. The brisk mountain air, birds chirping, and the excitement of the last leg of the Yellowstone adventure is too much for her to waste in the confines of the tent. Besides, today is to be the grandest part of the trip, what with the spectacular mountain lake and their first sighting of the Grand Tetons and their continuously snow-capped peaks. Jack snores to the crackling of the bacon, and wakes to her gentle tap of his shoulder, and whispering in his ear of "Rise and shine, sweetheart."

Soon he is sitting on the smooth rock sipping coffee, just a little irritated at Allyson's newfound early morning friskiness. Later, as they prepare to collapse the tent, she suggests, by soft caress, that the making of love is in the picture. Jack, never one to reject a romantic interlude, zips the tent tightly closed, and they share a sleeping bag. Their bodies and consciousness connect for the umpteenth time, and they are as close as physics and anatomy permit. During the pleasure, Jack has another realization: he and Allyson are really one. Jack knows that if not for love, he would be forever alone with his one-of-a-kind reality. As they share their own volcanic eruptions, losing themselves in the pleasure of it all, he wonders what people mean when they say they have a personal relationship with God. Flushed and sweaty, Jack knows that as long as he has the capability of love, he can truly be one with another. It would be hell on earth to be apart, alone, unloved. Now, he understands why symphony conductors lose themselves in music, rockers live to lose themselves in rock and roll, and race car drivers relish being one with their cars. Perhaps, he reflects as he slides from the sleeping bag, losing oneself is not a bad thing after all. Maybe a deathly riding companion is necessary for mortals to appreciate their consciousness.

There is a chill in the air as they exit the cloverleaf and cruise toward Fishing Bridge. Gray, billowing clouds hang from the sky and there is a hint of lightning crackling beyond pine-covered hilltops to their north. Allyson has assumed the lead and gears-down before leaning gracefully into the sharp curves. Jack, now with regained confidence, keeps up with her, smoothly gearing between first and fifth gears to the accompanying motorcycle power-purr. He revels in the sense of freedom and the rush of acceleration. Jack's unwanted Mammoth passenger is beginning to take more of a back seat on the journey.

Climbing a steep hill, Allyson points to her left and an idyllic lake with two swans impressively dancing a mating ritual. A small waterfall feeds the lake and hundreds of blossoming yellow and white mountain flowers dot the rocky shore. Cattails shoot up from a small floating island that, according to the informative sign, slowly migrates from shore to shore during the summer months. The smooth, glassy lake occasionally breaks its calm as a rainbow trout strikes above the surface for a hovering dragonfly or mosquito. Finally reaching the pinnacle of the mountain range, Allyson and Jack behold the great Yellowstone Lake, a natural wonder with miles and miles of forested shoreline nestled at the center of this preserved national jewel. Several small, rented motorboats transport eager fishers to the center of the huge lake and their seven-fish limit should rainbows and largemouths bite the barbless hooks.

As Jack and Allyson descend into a small enclave known as Grants Pass, gray billowing clouds begin to deposit their moisture, first in small, sparse drops, and soon as torrents of windy wet blankets. Allyson gives the hand signal to pull off the highway, and gradually comes to a stop on a gravel side road. Jack signals his intention to the car behind him, thankful for his wine-country prefix. Using his front brake on the slippery asphalt, he narrowly misses a porcupine darting across the road to safety. Jack reaches the side road, and sees a barely visible ancient railroad track laid during the roaring twenties. Unnerved by the narrow miss, Jack compares two-wheeler transportation to the safety of the rails, and for an instant, wishes he could take the train back to San Francisco. He briefly fantasizes about trains and the soothing clack, clack, clack of their rails.

Chapter 13

During Connie's final smoking break, she crushes her half-smoked cancer stick into the dirt, and announces to Clarence, and all others in earshot, that she is quitting the awful habit. Clarence, somewhat surprised at the announcement, asserts that he too is sick of smoking, and that it is starting to hurt his singing voice. He takes a nearly-new pack from his shirt pocket, crushes it in his hand, and tosses it into a trash can. At the elevator door while they wait, Connie wonders aloud what music they would be subjected to today, and if R414 will sing along. Clarence thinks that today Connie is uncharacteristically talkative, and perhaps she is high on caffeine. In the elevator, to a string quartet's rendition of "All You Need Is Love," Connie invites Clarence to her apartment for dinner. Surprised by the out-of-the-blue invitation, Clarence stutteringly accepts, and for the first time, sees the young ward clerk in a new light. He wonders what she sees in the likes of him, what with his dead-end job, struggling musician cliché, and chronic cash-flow problems. He also thinks her quite assertive for such a young woman. Connie is delighted that the orderly musician readily accepts her invitation of dinner, late-night coffee, and whatever else the cards may hold. She thinks to herself that sometimes a woman must take the lead in these matters.

The next day, Connie smiles at Clarence, who again is standing at the back of the reality orientation room, and their eyes briefly share the memory of their intimacy. R414 is decked out in smart jogging attire, with his gray hair carefully combed and gelled, and he sits fingering a plastic replica of the Golden Gate Bridge. In his eyes, you can see that he again is lost in terror-filled, paranoid thoughts. The serious therapist enters the room, and begins today's lesson by pinning several large head shots of people on the board. *Sharona points to the first one, and asks Jack to repeat after her: "Allyson."*

A Case of Severe Anterograde Amnesia

The brain scans showed the primary damage to Olive's brain was to the hippocampus. This structure, which resembles a sea horse, is found in the temporal lobes of the brain. It is critical for the formation of new memories, and scientists consider it a "gatekeeper" structure for new memory storage. Damage to the hippocampus is common in Alzheimer's disease, and it is particularly vulnerable to general oxygen deprivation such as occurs in some types of heart attacks, poisoning, and strokes. Olive suffered a rare but devastating stroke, resulting in severe anterograde amnesia. She could recall memories of events before the stroke, but could not transfer new ones from short-term to long-term storage. Consequently, Olive had no continuity from one experience to the next. When her attention would shift, she lost all memory of what happened previously.

At the food court of the large medical center there were three commercial fast-food restaurants, a Starbuck's, and a gift shop. They surrounded tables and booths accommodating visitors and patients, and it strangely resembled a shopping mall. At lunch, it was a busy center of activity for the hospital. The aroma of coffee, hamburgers, fries, tacos, and pizzas saturated the large room, and there was the ever-present clinking, clanging, and chatter typical of a large lunchroom. It was Olive's first outing to the food court, and she was accompanied by a therapist.

On the way to the food court, Olive was her usual busybody. With highly animated gestures, she commented on things of interest. She remarked the hall was narrow, "Don't you know." When passing someone, she would comment to them about her "flat in London," and "the children playing on the stoop."

"Let's put it in the boot" and "We'll walk to the top" were frequent, apparently random utterances. For weeks, the rehabilitation staff tried to find meaning in Olive's statements. That Olive was from London and visiting the United States when she suffered her stroke made it more difficult to decipher meaning. She appeared to be recalling memories from her youth that were prompted by current stimuli. Complicating the matter was that Olive had no relatives or friends with whom the medical staff could question about the meaning of her utterances. When they entered the food court, Olive, apparently stimulated by the aromas, asks the therapist if "lunch time for the children would include chips?"

The profound implications of anterograde amnesia on Olive's ability to function in society were made clear when she repeatedly ordered her lunch. Walking to the fast-food establishment, Olive studied the menu. When she reached the counter, she placed her order: "One hamburger and a soda." The young clerk asks if she would also like an order of fries. Olive answered, "No, thank you."

She turned to the therapist and asked if she was also going to order food. She then turned to the clerk, and said, "I would like a hamburger and a soda." Then, Olive turned to a person in the adjacent line, and made a comment to him about "children and a burning loft." Then, again, she turned to the confused clerk and said, "One hamburger, don't you know."

The clerk, becoming increasingly confused about the number of hamburgers being ordered, asked Olive if it was one or two hamburgers she was ordering. Olive calmly responded by saying, "We'll walk to the top."

Olive became distracted by a dropped tray behind her and turned to see the source of the noise. She then engaged the clerk's attention, and as if this was the first time they had interacted, asked if she could have a hamburger and a soda. Tragically for Olive, because of the anterograde amnesia, for her it was the first time she had placed the order. Eventually, they purchased the meal and Olive and the therapist sat at a small table in the food court. On the way out, Olive looked in the direction of the hamburger establishment and asked the therapist if they should order lunch for the children in the loft.

Past Tense

Chapter One

Most of us question our sanity at one time or another. In fact, I suspect those people who never question reality have the most tenuous connection to it. And because I suffered brain damage at birth, and endure this cerebral palsy as testimony to it, my connection with reality is especially suspect. Even I know that the neurons and chemistry of my brain are different, possibly rending my perceptions and consciousness flawed. I've heard of waking dreams, fugue states, dissociations, delusions, and hallucinations. I have also heard of Orson Wells, relativity, worm holes, and multidimensional space. And yes, with nerd resolve, I have seen each and every Star Trek episode ever made. So, I'm not only a geek, but a brain-damaged one to boot. With that said, Doctor, let me tell you about last Friday night and my experiences in the rare books section of the library.

My apologies for starting this story with such a worn-out cliché, but it really was a dark and dreary night. The clouds hung low, there were occasional dim flashes of light deep within them, and an ever-present chilly wind stirred the trees, bushes, and shrubs. Walking past the International Center and Bell Tower, I sensed that all was not well on this nighttime campus. I saw only two other people cutting through the starless night, walking rapidly to their cars, bundled tightly to reduce the chill. My only comfort on that early-spring night was the occasional blossoming lilac fragrance whisking past my nose, carried by the relentless wind. As I approached the library, it seemed that even its shadow was haunted by an infinite number of shadows. Occasionally, the moon would briefly find a small opening in the dark cloud cover, and for an instant, my moon shadow would appear only to quickly run and hide from this ominous night. I made my way to the library to the ever-present crippling cerebral palsy anthem: plop-slide, plop-slide, plop-slide. Plop, as one of my metal crutches slams the sidewalk, slide, as I drag my nearly-useless foot behind it. Then the other crutch plops, followed by the obedient slide. Plop-slide, plop-slide, plop-slide echoed above the rustling wind on that fateful Friday night. I finally reached the handicapped door and the large rectangular blue button to open it.

As the heavy glass door began its slow opening, I had my first encounter with déjà vu. Now Doctor, I am no stranger to waiting for the handicap doors to fully open, so my sense that this experience had just happened to me was not totally unexpected. Yet, this was more than a vague feeling, and more than a blurry recollection of something familiar. This déjà vu was the mother of all déjà vu, and I knew something was definitely awry in time. The sights, sounds, smells, and even the goose bumps raised on my arms by the chilly wind had, most certainly and vividly, just happened to me. I was reliving this moment in all its clarity. It was not some faint experience occurring in the not-so-distant past; it was here and almost now.

Yes, Doctor, we have all experienced déjà vu at some time in our lives, and to the scientists, it is a delay in processing time from one brain hemisphere to another, giving the illusion of pre-experience. To the mystics, it is proof of the metaphysical world and parallel universes. I certainly don't know the basis of déjà vu, but I do know that last Friday night, at the handicap door of the library, I had my first personal experience with the fabric of time and began questioning my perceptions of it. Finally, the sense of pre-experience dissolved as I plop-slid through the empty corridor of the library to the help desk, where a very serious middle-aged woman sat solitary and expressionless, eying my every gimpy movement.

"I would like a key to the rare books section," I said, showing her my faculty identification card. Actually, I said it three times as she tried to process my spastic speech: "You want tea in the bare foots rejection?"

Finally, with discomfort showing on her melancholy face, she gave me the swipe card and directions to the elevator that would take me to the bowels of the library, and my disturbing journeys back in time. Little did I know, as the elevator slowly made its way to that secluded place, I would relive the plight of the disabled, and the brutal mistreatment perpetrated on us.

After the ancient elevator groaned its way to the lowest basement floor of the library, the doors parted to a sign reading: Rare Books. Turning right, I followed a black arrow pointing the way to two large metal doors and a swipe card box that would open them. Balancing myself on one of my metal canes while the other one swung from my wrist, I swiped the card through the receptacle and a blue light flashed, granting me access. Again balancing myself on one of my metal crutches, I was able to wedge myself through the ponderous doors, and into the musty archive of old and precious books. The metal doors slammed closed behind me, and I was left standing alone in the dim light. Apparently, the Americans with Disabilities Act had yet to reach into the depths of this university library to provide me, and my kind, with unobstructed access to its most valued books.

The rare books section of the library was a lot smaller than I had anticipated. There were five floor-to-ceiling book racks and two glass enclosed bookcases with finely controlled temperature and humidity. The windowless room was illuminated only by flickering florescent tubes accompanied by a constant hum. The cement walls were painted some drab off-white color, and the ceiling was constructed of acoustic tiles. The carpeted floor of the room muffled my every plop-slide as I made my way to the first bookshelf. The legend on the wall listed the books alphabetically by author and title.

I scanned the list and found Freud, Sigmund, and a 1908 treatise on personality and eroticism. I pulled that dusty book from the shelf, and plop-slid to a small wooden table. Leaning my metal crutches on an adjacent chair, I sat down to peruse the first edition.

When I opened the book, I was overcome by another bout of déjà vu, only this time it did not stop as abruptly as it came on. I felt lightheaded, and the room began to spin, first in slow spirals, and then faster and faster until the walls and bookcases became a Navajo White blur. The room became unrecognizable as the spinning increased, and my body seemed to be lifted higher and higher and then, remarkably, through the ceiling, upward floor-by-floor, until I was looking down on the building. I could clearly see the library's roof and barely lit rectangular windows through that dark and dreary night. The library became smaller and smaller as I continued to be lifted by some invisible, indefinable force. I could see the grassy expanse surrounding the large building, the fountains and budding trees become minuscule landscaping, and the campus itself shrink smaller and smaller, and then, suddenly, I saw and felt an explosion of light and energy.

London, England
November 19, 1888
7:15 a.m.

The damp wind cuts through his tattered, well-worn rag of a coat, and Ben shivers uncontrollably in the corner of the shanty. Long ago separated from his mother, uncle, grandmother, and sisters, he fends for himself by seeking shelter with prostitutes. During the day, he relies on the kindness of strangers on street corners for coins and scraps of food dropped in his cap.

Handicapped at birth by crippling paralysis, his poverty-stricken family did their best to feed and clothe him when he was young. When Ben grew into a deformed young man with barely intelligible slurred speech, he decided he would no longer burden them, so migrated to the city for the employment he hoped would be forthcoming. What Ben did not anticipate was the hatred and fear he evoked in some who blindly held him responsible for the death ravaging this dirty, dank, desperate city. Last week, his friend, lover, and protector, Mary Jane Kelly, had become another victim of the Whitechapel Murderer, a sinister killer who prowled the nights of east London and preyed on its downtrodden.

That Ben survived birth was either a miracle or a curse, depending on the hunger he felt deep in his stomach and the chill penetrating to the core of his body. His family farmed a small plot of fertile soil several miles from London, providing fresh potatoes, beans, corn, and tomatoes. The excess milk and produce they took to the open market

69

helped them barter or buy the other necessities of life. Ben was a difficult birth. The midwives did all they could to hasten his passage through the birth canal, but Ben was breech and eventually, nature took its course. He was slow to respond to the sharp slaps to his bare bottom, but finally cried weakly to his worldly arrival. For several days his mother tried nursing him, but he was rigid in her arms and could barely suck enough breast milk to sustain him. Ben's mother supplemented his diet with goats' milk carefully spooned into his mouth. Still, Ben seemed to have a strong survival instinct, one he would need throughout his handicapped life as a street urchin and beggar.

As a youth, there was precious little time for boyish games, what with the daily business of survival. Though the farm was small, it took the sunrise-to-sunset energy of all in the extended family to scratch out an existence. The small farmhouse sheltered the seven family members, and the large fireplace warmed it on cold winter nights. Ben's father died shortly after his birth from one of the diseases that periodically swept the nearby village and surrounding farms. Ben's uncle moved in thereafter to help the family pull through, and did much of the farming and milking. When Ben was four, he was given small wooden crutches with rags serving as cushions for his underarms. He could manage his spastic body by slowly dragging his feet through the dirt, mud, and occasional snow. As he grew taller, so did the crutches. Slow to talk, formal schooling was out-of-the-question, but his mother and oldest sister helped him learn the basics of reading and writing.

His speech was distorted, often making him the butt of jokes for the townspeople. When he passed the local tavern on shopping trips with his mother, the drunkards imitated his speech and made unkind comments. His mother held him close to her and reminded him that the boisterous lot of ne'er-do-wells, layabouts, and slack-jaws were crippled by addiction to alcohol. By the time he was ten, his mates and townspeople called him "Crip" and few weeks went by where he was not bullied and beaten by school children whenever he ventured beyond the sanctuary of his home and farm. Fortunately, Ben was born into a loving and nurturing family, poor though they were. He was a hard worker, and during his youth worked shoulder-to-shoulder with his uncle trying to do chores as well as any able-bodied man. It certainly took more time for him to complete the job, and even longer to talk about it, but Ben was not short of energy and determination.

When Ben turned seventeen he decided to strike out on his own, to become his own man, to embrace his future and whatever it might bring. He was tired of working long hours on the farm, but more than anything, he loathed the social isolation. Most of his time was spent with family, and when he ventured into town, he always found rejection. He suspected the townspeople were narrow-minded and rigid-thinkers, and that London, the large urban center ripe with culture and sophistication, would hold more opportunities for work and a social life. Like most young men of his age, Ben's thoughts often turned to women and companionship. Yet unlike most men of Ben's age, he knew the likelihood of finding a woman accepting of him and his disabilities were slim at best. Never one to be intimidated by poor odds, Ben bid his family farewell amid crying, hugs, and a manly handshake from his uncle. Early one morning, he caught a ride in a horse-drawn cart and shared the odoriferous accommodations with a gaggle of geese. By late evening, Ben was deposited in the east end of London and spent the night crouched in an alleyway. He awoke to the chatter of alley-dwellers bemoaning death at the hands of England's notorious "Jack the Ripper" and murder most savage. Apparently, a woman of the night, "Dark Annie," was found on the cobblestones hacked to death not far from Ben's nightly respite.

Ben was nearly overwhelmed by London. Nothing at his home or in the small village prepared him for the sights, sounds, and smells of this huge city. He spent most of his first day wandering throughout the eastern part of the city, watching people bargain, argue, boast, and attend to commerce. Street hustlers seemed permanent fixtures trying to beg, borrow, or steal from the urbanites. The well-to-do society, smartly dressed and barking orders to servants, traveled in horse drawn taxis, never giving Ben a second glance. Smoke, dust, and flies filled the air, as did an ever-present stench of horse, mule, and donkey droppings. That first day in London, Ben bought bread and potatoes from a street vendor and washed them down with water from a horse trough. His spastic speech muscles also made chewing and swallowing difficult, and he took care to take small bites. Ben knew he must carefully apportion his money, generously given to him by his mother and uncle, until he could find employment and begin the business of fending for him self. By nightfall, Ben was tired and more than just a little fearful of what the darkness would bring. He found a place behind a stable, and slept lightly between large piles of dung and straw, awaking several times to shouts, cries, and laughter of a city that appeared never to sleep. During the night, a sense of loneliness befell him, like a dark melancholy blanket, and for the first time since bidding his family farewell, Ben had a crisis of confidence. What terrible mistake had he made in leaving the bosom of his loving family?

For Ben, the third day of independence was as frightening and depressing as the previous ones. Several times Ben approached people for jobs, but rarely would they even stop to talk to him. The first outright rejection came from a pub owner who laughed aloud when Ben asked if he needed dishwashing and spittoon dumping. "Off you go, Crip" he said to Ben while gesturing with a sweeping motion with his hand, clearly not wanting to waste time with the likes of him. No stranger to rejection, Ben still felt a tightness in his stomach at the dismissal— a combination of anger and despair. The second rejection, even worse than the first, came from a kindly elderly woman at a boarding house. Ben approached her at the rear of the structure while she dumped bath water in the street, and he asked several times if a servant position was available. He tried to convey that he would be happy to work dawn-to-dusk for meals and a cot. The woman was unable to understand his distorted speech, try as she may. Finally, in frustration, she placed a coin in his spastic hand and said, "Now I've business to attend, let me on with my drudgery." She patted him on the cheek and went into the boarding house carrying the empty wooden pail. For Ben, rejection was devastating enough without the added pity. Nevertheless, he placed the generous offering in his coin purse for safekeeping. The worst of London times happened that night when Ben was mugged and beaten by two drunks who took his coin purse and shoes.

The assault came out of the blue; the two assailants pounced on Ben with vehemence and ferocity, and a determination to kill for the meager bounty in his purse. Reeking of rum, they were clumsy, brutal, and effective in their thievery. While one kicked Ben about the head and neck, and clubbed him with his crutch, the other rummaged through his pockets and belongings for valuables. Ben tried to fight back, but was outnumbered and outmatched. One thief, a heavyset, unwashed drunk was most malicious in the assault, and spat on Ben's bloodied unconscious body when finally the kicking and beating ended. Laughing, singing, and impervious to the morality of beating senseless a disabled person, they stumbled through the alley looking for yet another unfortunate victim. As the sun peeked over the smoky rooftops of the uncaring city, Ben gradually came to, moaning in despair, and groaning in pain. Then, an angel of the night knelt beside him, blotted blood from his brow, and said: "Lie quiet, lad."

Ben managed to open his eyes through swollen brows, and tried to utter gratitude to Mary Jane Kelly. She helped Ben stand, and carrying his crutches, took him to her home, a small lean-to shanty she shared with other women of the night.

Ben slept for nearly twenty hours, and only occasionally awoke to the tender nursing of Mary Jane. Mary Jane Kelly, an Irish girl just-turned twenty-five, migrated to London several years earlier for the same reasons that prompted Ben to leave farm and family: to seek independence and begin the business of living. Sadly, Mary Jane fell on hard times when her employment as a chamber maid abruptly ended with the death of her mistress. She settled in the east end of London with several other women on the out, and soon found comfort and solace in drinking and pubs. Men were eager to buy food and beer for the pretty young thing, and eventually began depositing pound and pence on her night stand for her favors. Like most women practicing the oldest profession, she never consciously made the decision to become a prostitute, but fell into the dangerous work over time and as a consequence of circumstances.

When Mary Jane saw the crippled youngster lying in the alley bloodied and beaten, she automatically came to his aid, not because of guilt should she not, but because his pathetic sight so tugged at her heartstrings. Despite the hopelessness of her life, Mary Jane was good at heart, and steadfastly cared for Ben until his body healed and strength returned. Over time, Ben and Mary Jane found companionship, comfort, and camaraderie in each other's company and arms.

Several women shared the lean-to shanty, and it was an unwritten rule that no Jacks were to be brought there. The shanty was sparse, but it was home for the women, and a safe respite from their dangerous profession. They cooked on a makeshift wood stove that also provided warmth on cold London nights. Mary Jane had a sleeping cot, but most of the women slept on bedrolls carefully aligned on the wood floor. The accommodation was always clean and strangely comfortable given the comings and goings at all hours. Mary Jane gave Ben her cot during his lengthy recuperation, and she slept quietly on the floor beside him. As he got stronger, he told her of his life and dreams, and she shared with him her goal of a flower stand and breaking away from this decrepit existence.

Mary Jane showed talent in understanding Ben's spastic speech, and rarely required repetitions. Eventually, they took walks during the day, and Mary Jane was patient at Ben's slowness. She never did for him things he was capable of doing, and seemed to have an understanding of the importance of self-reliance. They shared a camaraderie cemented by their bodies. While Ben's body was nearly useless, Mary Jane's body was, as she described it, a temporary asset. After a few months, Mary Jane and the Crip, as their neighbors called them, became a common fixture on the streets of London.

Neither Ben nor Mary Jane had ever felt truly romantically loved, and their union, strange though it was, was the very best of times for them. The world they shared was like a loving bubble protecting and insulating them from the scorn, ridicule, and hatred of London's proper citizenry. To the city's upper crust, Mary Jane was a woman of the street pandering to its most decadent needs. Ben was a most pitiful creature, the very sight of him creating discomfort and dread. They were both society's throwaways, useless street trash festering of disability, disease, and death. Several times on their daily jaunts, they retreated to the safety of the shanty-home when the good people of London threw stones at them. They were accused of everything from being Satan's messengers to harbingers of the deadly disease that ravaged the city. Most dreaded in the hearts of Londoners was that the evil two would procreate and bring a new generation of wickedness to the city.

Ben saw Mary Jane as an accepting woman, oblivious to his twisted, feeble body and savvy to his distorted speech. It was as though she had a blind spot to his infirmities and connected with him on a deeper, more important level. Her beauty mesmerized him. That Mary Jane sold her body to strangers was understandably disturbing to Ben, but on a deeper level, he too understood the realities of her life. Starvation and death, or even worse, scavenging for scraps of food with the ferals and rats, were the only alternatives available to Mary Jane should she not sell her body. And the rum she drank to excess helped deaden the nightly ordeals. Ben and Mary Jane both lived for the future where they could get honorable employment and live respectable lives. Their dream was not to amass great wealth and possessions; it was simply to live a life together basking in love and companionship, and live in a world where their bodies were relegated to the shadows. Tragically, the Whitechapel Murderer, or Jack the Ripper as the locals called him, savagely took Mary Jane from Ben late one chilly autumn night in a dank alleyway.

It was a typical night for Ben and Mary Jane, at least as typical as it could be given the goings-on of the residents of the shanty. Ben returned from job-hunting at dusk, again spending long hours confronting rejection, ridicule, and scorn. Earlier that evening, a large communal crock of porridge had been made, and Ben enjoyed spooning it into his bowl and feasting on the hot, thin liquid. Mary Jane had left earlier that evening, and Ben missed the cheek-peck she often gave him as she bid him nightly farewell. Exhausted from his daily toil, Ben slept soundly on the cot awaiting Mary Jane's return. Early the next morning, Ben arose in near-panic when he realized Mary Jane had not returned to the shanty. Near-panic became true-panic when the alleyway again resonated with the chatter, gabble, and tattle of Jack the Ripper's recent savagery. Only this time, Ben's worst fears would be realized: the Ripper's latest victim was Mary Jane Kelly.

When Ben approached Mary Jane's body lying on cobblestones not far from the pub she frequented, he screamed in pain and despair, and knelt beside her, his crutches falling into blood-puddles. He cradled her lifeless body, asking "Why, Why, Why?"

Several Bobbies pulled him from her, his clothes stained by her blood, hands dripping the still-warm liquid. He fell into a heap at their feet. Sobbing uncontrollably, Ben slowly made his way back to the shanty, packed his belongings into his worn carpetbag, and hobbled through the uncaring crowd of early-risers, oblivious to their ever-present mean slurs on him and his kind. He sat sobbing on a quiet corner, his crippled feet tucked beneath his body, more alone than he had ever been. As an elderly woman passed him, she dropped a crust of hard bread into the cap lying next to him. He heard her remark to her male companion as they continued on their way: "Disgraceful. Why don't the likes of 'em find work and some decency?"

Then, almost as godly reprieve from his pain, the morning began spinning, first slowly, then more rapidly, and as it gained speed and momentum. I was gradually lifted higher and higher above the smoky street corner, elevated farther into the early dawn until the streets and alleys became small networks of spider webs, then the city merely a dot on an island, and as I shot upward, I experienced another explosion of light and energy. I found myself again in the rare books section of the library wondering if it was a dream or a hallucination.

Well Doctor, what I witnessed was as real as you, this room, and the sounds of the chirping birds just outside this window. I not only witnessed Ben's ordeal from some ethereal vantage point just above him, but I felt as he felt, heard what he heard, smelled what he smelled, saw through his eyes, and experienced the depth of his despair. So Doctor, I leave it to you to decide my fate? Was it a dream? A hallucination? Am I psychotic and in need of institutionalization? Help me, Doctor.

The Peyote Way*

"The Peyote Way" was originally published in *The Family Guide to Surviving Stroke and Communication Disorders* (2nd edition) (Jones and Bartlett Publishers).

There is no shortage of missionaries on the Navajo Indian Reservation, and they can be very persuasive. Many of Earnest's clan converted to Christian religions of various denominations, and it seemed fewer and fewer of his people were members of the Native American Church. For Earnest, it was sad that so few people spoke Navajo, lived in Hogans, and had a connection to the roots of the noble Dine' people with such a remarkable history. He spent his life on this huge reservation, tending to his herd of sheep, growing corn, and raising a large family. Even after the death of his wife, Earnest refused to move from his beloved Hogan to one of the government track housing units in Kayenta, Arizona. His traditional Hogan, with the door facing magnificent sunrises, sits atop a plateau with a panoramic view of Monument Valley and the commanding red rock formations.

Earnest was a traditional Navajo and proud of it. At 77 years of age, Earnest prided himself on being a hard worker and a fine carpenter. One day while helping a relative shingle a tool shed, Earnest slipped from the ladder and fell to the ground, hitting his head on a large rock. He was rushed to Farmington, New Mexico where doctors stopped the bleeding inside of his brain and saved his life. The fall from the ladder caused aphasia and weakness on the right side of his body. After three weeks in the rehabilitation unit, Earnest's family arranged a healing ceremony and obtained a weekend pass from the hospital. The miracle of modern medicine would be supplemented by the Peyote Way.

It was challenging for the English-speaking examiner to evaluate Earnest's aphasia. There are very few Navajo speech-language pathologists, and even fewer who are bilingual, so the evaluation session required an interpreter. During the evaluation, Earnest was cooperative, polite, and in true traditional Dine' way, soft-spoken, and lacking of eye-contact. Several times he would gesture by using his lips and chin to show the general location of an object. His youngest daughter, a student at Dine' College, was fluent in Navajo and English. However, several times during the evaluation it was necessary to adjust the assessment protocol to adapt to the unique nature of the Navajo language. For example, when testing for anomia, the examiner asked Earnest to look at several photographs and provide the names of relatives, expecting the interpreter to say, "He said that was 'Robert' or 'Lucy' or 'Ruby.'" However, the interpreter explained Earnest would say their relationship in the family or clan, rather than their names— a common way for traditional Navajos to refer to relatives. Another adjustment had to be made for the tonal nature of Navajo because it appeared Earnest was perseverating on a grandchild's name. When shown a picture of one grandchild, he appeared to be repeating the same name immediately after being shown a picture of another child. The interpreter noted their names were very similar phonemically, and that it was primarily the pitch rise and fall on the final vowels of their names that signaled different children. Earnest appeared to benefit from therapies, but there was heavy reliance on the interpreter who attended each session. There were inherent difficulties in quantifying gains and structuring treatment because of the language issues.

The Navajo Indian Reservation extends into Arizona, New Mexico, and Utah, and the Peyote Healing Ceremony was held in a remote region of its eastern border. It is called the "checkerboard area" because private and reservation lands appear checked on a map. The large eight-sided wood Hogan with its east-facing door easily accommodated the churchgoers for the all-night ceremony. Earnest eagerly anticipated the religious service, and when the time came, he sat at a place of honor in front of the congregation.

When the church members entered the Hogan, they walked around the interior in a clockwise manner, symbolizing a person's travel from birth to death. They greeted Earnest and sat cross-legged in a circle on blankets or sheepskins. The "Healing Way" ceremony lasted for nearly 14 hours, with a wood stove providing heat for the 24 churchgoers. Coals were taken from the wood stove and placed on the ground, and throughout the ceremony cedar chips were placed on them to produce the sweet-smelling smoke that served as a purifying agent. The services were conducted in Navajo by a special medicine man, a "Roadman," holding high esteem in the community. At the beginning of the ceremony the Roadman explained the purpose behind it. He said Earnest's communication disorder was caused by him falling out of harmony with nature. On the floor of the Hogan, a mound of dirt was formed into a quarter-circle called a "moon circle" that represented Earnest's life travel. A peyote cactus button was placed on the moon circle to represent his place on the road of life. The peyote used by the participants in the ceremony was provided as a powder and placed in a tea. The container of peyote tea was placed next to the moon circle and taken by the church members four or five times during the ceremony. The use of the peyote cactus among some Navajo Indians is an important element of their religious and healing beliefs. The drug mescaline, a stimulant and hallucinogenic, is derived from peyote, and is associated with taking God into the body. To believers, peyote helps transform them into a state of physical, mental, and spiritual well-being and helps make the Great Spirit and other supernatural forces more apparent.

During the service, prayers sung in Navajo were offered by members of the Church and directed at the Great Spirit and lesser Gods for the benefit of the patient. The idea was to coax them into helping Earnest again become one with nature to cure his aphasia. Hand-rolled tobacco-mix cigarettes were used as a medium through which the words were conveyed by the smoke to the Great Spirit. A flute signaled to the Gods that prayers were forthcoming, and there was singing of traditional Native American songs accompanied by the rhythmic beat of several drums and rattles. Church members sang in perfect harmony. The prayers were sincere efforts by Earnest's friends and family to persuade the Great Spirit to help him. That cold winter night in a remote region of the Navajo Indian Reservation, the ancient songs, rattles and flutes, drum beats, and prayers resonated throughout the enchanting high desert plateau, and Earnest basked in the traditional Navajo way. The ceremony ended at sunrise with the congregation singing the beautiful "Morning Song." For breakfast, several large bowls of traditional Navajo food were served communal style to the members. As the faithful left for their homes, Earnest and his family thanked them for their attendance and bid them farewell.

As with all religious customs and rituals, it was difficult objectively to assess the result of the Peyote Healing Ceremony on the patient's speech and language abilities. At the conclusion of the ceremony, there was no demonstrable improvement in his communication abilities. However, there was a dramatic change in Earnest's adjustment to the aphasia. He was much more positive about his illness and the depression he was experiencing appeared to lift. On Monday, Earnest returned to the rehabilitation unit and continued the therapies.

*What is reported here does not divulge sacred rites of the Native American Church. Permissions were obtained for a nonmember observer, and there was a representative from tribal government present to ensure appropriate witnessing and reporting of the ceremony.

"Murder Challenged" was originally published in *The Psychology of Neurogenic Communication Disorders: A Primer for Health Care Professionals* (Pearson Allyn & Bacon Publishers).

You see us in airports, malls, movie theaters, and on sidewalks. You hear us talk in restaurants, schools and churches. But you don't really see us. You don't really hear us. We're like a flutter on the outskirts of your senses. You've been taught not to stare, not to be nosy. When you're forced to acknowledge us, you become nervous, awkward. You speak slowly and loudly. You get very sincere looks on your faces. We're alien to you, and you don't know how to act. You don't know what to say, or how to say it.

Oh, I'm not saying you are mean or rude. For the most part, you're not. You just feel uncomfortable around us. Hell, that's understandable. We often feel uncomfortable around you. A long time ago, I began to understand why this happens. I think it is because we're not just different, we're defective, and we're defective in so many different ways. It is frightening to know that our defects could easily have happened, or might still, happen to you. This can be scary, and being scared is the worst type of discomfort.

We, the physically and mentally disabled, live in a different world from yours. Ours is a world of shadows where real participation in yours has been prohibited by God, abnormal genes, birth defects, brain injuries, and spastic muscles. We live on the outskirts of reality town, and we rarely visit Main Street.

Chapter 1

My name is Ben. I'm one of those aliens to your world. I have been one since birth and I was a big disappointment to my parents. According to the doctors, I was "stressed" during the birth process. Precious molecules of oxygen didn't get to parts of my brain. The result is me and a disorder known as cerebral palsy. You probably know me as

"Spaz," "Retard," "Gimp," or "Crip." Those were labels given to me by my brother, and hordes of playground bullies. I'm defective because the muscles of my legs, arms, and speech are always tightly pulling against themselves. I spend a lot of time working against myself.

Oh, I'm not mentally deficient. In fact, I have a tested I.Q. that is higher than most, or as they say in statistics, one standard deviation above the norm. My intelligence surprises most people. They just can't accept the fact that I'm not mentally retarded. I suppose it is because I don't appear intelligent. Spastic muscles make my movements slow and awkward. Seeing me shuffle down a concrete sidewalk makes people think my defects include concrete thinking.

It's my speech that throws most listeners for a loop. Because of those spastic muscles, my talking is labored and distorted, and it really does sound retarded. After hearing me for the first time, almost all listeners respond with slowly spoken, one-word-at-a-time, replies. You know what I'm talking about, the kind of speech reserved for three-year-olds. It's kind of ironic that I'm usually superior in intelligence and education to those talking down to me. Over the years, I've purposefully learned a super vocabulary. I like to see the facial expressions when I say something like, "I'm perplexed with the graphic illustrations of the location of some of the mall's stores," or ask, "Do you know the shortest distance to the electronics establishment?"

It's fun to see the conflicts on the listeners' faces. I can almost hear what they're thinking. "How can this be? A retard using complex words? Is this candid camera?" People really get conflicted when, on the first day of class, I walk into the large, auditorium classroom and take my place at the podium. I'm sure some of the students think some retard got confused, accidentally wandered into a university classroom, and some kindly aide will soon remove the creature.

I have had a lot of speech therapy to help me sound more "normal." Quite frankly, I'm sick of all the therapies. As I told Janet, my girlfriend, I've had enough therapy to make a hog puke. Why can't people just accept my "spastic dysarthria," as the medical types call it, as a different dialect or accent? I've heard people from New Orleans and Liverpool, and my accent isn't really much more unusual. Oh well, I'm not a linguist or a social worker. Things are just the way they are and I'll never be able to change them.

Janet is a very unusual woman. We've been together for almost five years and I must say, she is something special, and I don't mean "special" in the way people refer to me. I still can't understand why she was ever attracted to me, and each day of my life, I wonder why she stays with me. We've lived together for three years in this small, one bedroom house, not far from her office where she labors with other defectives. She was recently promoted to some type of vocational coordinator and spends a lot of time finding "sheltered" work for the disabled. Janet is good at what she does and she seems to enjoy it.

Janet isn't one of us. In fact, her body and mind are remarkably flawless. She turned thirty last month, which I noted is fairly old for a woman (this comment was met by her displaying her middle finger in my direction). To undo that unsuccessful attempt at humor, I commented that she has the "aging gracefully" gene. Her jet black hair is void of even one strand of gray, and her skin is as white and smooth as the day she was born. She has long, slender legs, and trophy breasts, which appear impervious to gravity. Although she complains of being too fat, she is not overweight. Oh, I'm sure that in the world of skinny super models, where lunch is glass of water and Saltine (no wonder they always have sour looks on their faces), she would be considered overweight, but in the real world, she is just fine. I appreciate her for what she is. She was blessed with normal limbs, muscles, and a functional brain. As far as I'm concerned she only has one flaw. She appears to have a blind spot. I don't think she sees the defects in me or her clients at work. I wonder if she even perceives us as having flaws. Janet is a very unusual woman, all right.

I'll never forget the first time we met. It was in a course I audited, just for the fun of it, titled, "The Psychology of Disabilities," which was taught in the evenings by a very normal, middle-aged woman with a degree in psychology. I'll admit, I kind of resented her postulating the psychological effects of disabilities without ever having limped a mile in our shoes. Apparently, we suffer from everything from denial to repressed anger. Some of her ideas were good, but others were pretty lame, at least from my perspective. When some of the more vocal students confronted the professor about her personal lack of knowledge about disabilities, she defended herself by noting that you don't have to have a baby to be a good pediatrician, or that giving birth to one doesn't make you an obstetrician. True enough. However, her defense was not good enough for the rest of the disabled in the class, and there were a lot of them. There were quite a few comments about why the university couldn't find a disabled psychologist to teach the class, what with this being the era of affirmative action and all. The good professor managed to fend off the remainder of the attacks, and regain control of the class, until she broached the subject of what to call us. That's when the good professor lost control.

It might not seem a big deal to you, but to the disabled, what we are labeled is important. I suppose a label is big deal to a lot of people, disabled or not. After all, would a doctor want to be called a nurse, or a bricklayer a carpenter? Nowadays, there are a lot of words which set off politically correct debates: Black, Hispanic, Oriental, right-wing, Gay. Are the meanings of the words "Colored People" substantially different from "People of Color?" Reasonable or not, these words cause reactions in people. Among the disabled, the semantic reactions occur over words like "Disabled," "Handicapped," "Special,""Alternately Abled," and "Challenged." They set off strong emotions, and sometimes I think countries have gone to war for less. Personally, I don't understand all the hubbub. People should be able to call themselves anything they want as long as it accurately defines them. I prefer to call myself "defective." I am, you know, and no word in English, or any other language, can hide or even minimize that fact. Unfortunately, I don't see many other disabled people rushing to use my word. When I offered it to the class, Janet and I began.

I was brutally attacked by almost the entire class, including the professor. "How could I be so insensitive?" one person asked. "Why not just call us scum?" agreed another. "It only focuses on the negative!" a third student asserted.

Surprised at the heated response from the students, I sat down to lick my wounds when a voice from a wheelchair said, "Shame on you," clearly the work of a speech synthesizer. One student suggested I be expelled from the class and there was a hum of general agreement. Geez, what was their problem? Had I not been disabled, I think they would have clubbed me with canes and pinned me to the wall with their wheelchairs.

So, I sat there while the anger saturated the room. My face was flushed and I felt rather embarrassed. Then, Janet spoke. She proceeded to give an eloquent speech in defense of me. Her point was that, although she didn't like the word "defective" to describe people, I had a right to call myself anything I wanted. And who were they to castigate me and my vocabulary. She concluded her Patrick Henry defense of me with the idea that in their politically correct frenzy, they forgot I have freedom of speech regardless of how uncomfortable it made them feel. Their uncomfortable feelings were not a sufficient reason to trash the Bill of Rights, or to deprive me of my God-given right of expression. Who said college should always be comfortable? Then, she sat down, and the professor finally gained control of the classroom.

After class, I made for a quick exit. Behind me, I could see hordes of angry alternately-abled fascists swarming toward me. I was more than a little frightened. I knew they wanted to finish the business started earlier in the class. All I wanted was to escape to my small apartment, swill a beer or two, and try to forget the nightmare that was this class. Thank God, easy egress for the handicapped was not a reality, despite the American's With Disabilities Act. I managed to outrun the angry hordes. I saw them moving slowly behind me, torches and pitch forks held high, while speech synthesizers droned: "Kill him, Hang him." Well, maybe it wasn't exactly like that, but it was quite a sight nonetheless.

It was a short walk to my apartment and it was a beautiful autumn evening. Looking behind me, I could see that the mob of politically correct McCarthy's had lost my trail, and that I might have time for a fancy coffee. I ducked into a fashionable coffee shop for a decaffeinated Latte. As usual, the line was long. There is no such thing as a quick cup of espresso. I patiently stood there awaiting my turn, when I heard someone say to me, "I see you got out alive." I turned and there was Janet, and I was forever smitten. I said something to the effect that the class's response to me was "much ado about nothing," and she agreed. I also pushed Shakespeare a bit further with a comment about a rose (or stinkweed) by any other name. I thanked her for coming to my defense, even though I was perfectly capable of it, had I not been so startled by their anger. She graciously accepted my qualified thanks, and we sat together at one of those miniature tables seen in coffee shops around the world. For the next couple of hours we talked, discussed, argued, and laughed. I learned about her and she about me. It was one of the most satisfying two hours of my life. As we left the coffee shop, I had her telephone number firmly tucked away in my wallet.

About two days later, I mustered the courage to call Janet. I was going to wait longer, say three or four days, but I was too caught up in the excitement of possibilities. So, I ran the risk of appearing too eager, rang her up, as they say in England, and was both surprised and delighted when she accepted my proposition of a movie and dinner. Actually, after the phone call, I felt a little disappointed. Janet so readily accepted my invitation, and so eagerly agreed to go out with me, that I began to wonder what was wrong with her. What major personality flaw did she have? What kind of woman would be so eager to go out with a defective like me? I'm painfully aware that I'm not the most attractive man in the world what with my spastic muscles and all. And even if my muscles would relax, I'm still not blessed with the features most women swoon over.

And then there is my personality. I never bought into the idea that just because my passage through my mother's birth canal was a major headache, I should forever be humble, quiet and reserved in thought and actions. I was never the kind to sit quietly on the outskirts, and to know my place in normal society. Quite frankly, I adopted the attitude at an early age: "Screw the huddled masses and their superior, self-righteous beliefs about me and my kind." I simply believe that even with my defects, I'm as good as or better than most. I also don't take life and disabilities so seriously. I usually see the humorous side of most things, and that includes the world of the handicapped. I have been called a "spastic with an attitude." So, given my obvious physical flaws and not so obvious personality ones, I was, at first, disappointed at Janet for agreeing to go out with someone like me. I would have to examine her very closely for fatal feminine flaws.

Luckily, I am able to drive my specially equipped van. It's quite a machine. I have easy access to the steering apparatus and other essential control systems, including my state-of-the-art stereo system. The van didn't need major modifications. It cost a pretty penny, but it is well worth it. I purposefully chose the brightest red color, fanciest wheels, and a 440 cubic inch powerhouse because I wanted it to be more of a rod than some dark, dreary machine you see at handicapped parking spaces. Last year, I had dual glass packed mufflers put on. I just love to hear the engine start. I swear it growls, like an angry lion with a bad case of hemorrhoids. I know, I'm a little long in the tooth to be excited about mufflers and engines, but I suppose if I can have arrested development, it can include this teenage fancy for big engines and loud mufflers.

Janet was impressed with the rod all right. I think she was a little surprised, too. Where did I get the money for tuck and roll leather seats, oversized tires, and all of the other options and accessories? She knew I was a professor on campus, and I'm also certain she knew that professors, especially third year assistant ones like me, didn't make big bucks.

I don't tell people I am a published novelist, a writer of mysteries. I even write them under a pseudonym. When I say I'm published, I mean I have had two books actually hit the bookstores. My first book, *Murder in Montana*, didn't quite shake the world of publishing with its sales. Sixteen hundred books were sold and most of them to libraries. Didn't quite hit the *New York Times* best sellers list with my first try. But my second book, *A Death in Denver*, surprised me and my publisher, who I think only published my books because I'm disabled, a kind of politically correct novelty act that can be boasted about in corporate meetings. But, surprise, surprise, as Gomer Pyle would say, I sold over a hundred thousand copies of my second book. It's now in its third printing, and twice a year, I get rewarded handsomely for it. I get 10% of the net sales, minus returns, for the first 10,000 copies, and 12% for any books sold beyond that. So I get a couple bucks for each book, and when you sell thousands of them, it adds up. My van was the first purchase I made with the royalty checks.

As planned, Janet and I had our first real date. The movie was yet another coming of age sophomore romp where teenage boys desperately and clumsily seek their first sexual experience. Although the plot was predictable, and the bathroom humor only marginally laughable, we had a wonderful time. Janet alternately laughed and was disgusted at the appropriate times. We ordered the same meal at dinner, which was the required first-date fare of a northern Italian plate of fishy pasta with a pretentious name and too much garlic. Although our first date was less than unique, we enjoyed ourselves with easy conversation and comfortable interaction. Never did I detect the slightest aversion to my physical and speech defects and, in fact, Janet initiated the always awkward good night kiss. Sadly, there was no invitation to late night coffee-sex in her apartment, but the kiss alone sustained me. Driving home, I knew I had met the woman of my dreams, one I would pursue until I was thoroughly rejected.

During the fall semester, we shared more sophomore movies, pasta plates, and awkward kisses. I grew to love everything about her: her perfume, hair, skin, voice, smile, walk. I was hopelessly mesmerized by this wonderful, strange creature who accepted me for me. We met for coffee, walked along the Oak River, and talked and talked on the telephone and via e-mail. Once, while standing in line at "our" coffee shop, we both overheard a seven-year-old girl ask her mother why I walked and talked so funny. Of course, I have heard questions and comments like these almost daily since I was old enough to understand them. I have learned to ignore most of them, and for the hurtful ones, I have rationalized them. I was delighted when Janet appeared either to immediately forget the comment or to ignore it all together. She appeared to have the indifferent, thick-skinned attitude necessary if she were to spend more time with me. I knew as long as we were together, there would be many more comments. To respond to them is simply a waste of time and energy. Nothing will ever stop them, so all I can do is control my reactions, which I'm getting very good at. I am almost impervious to them.

People don't like talking about sex and the disabled. Hell, most people won't even allow themselves to think about it, although our society is preoccupied with sex. It permeates our movies, books, and television shows. Old people remember it, and the young ones can't talk about anything else. Our billboards, magazine ads, and television snippets use it to sell us everything from tires to toilet paper. But you never see sex and the disabled together. Society would rather think of us as asexual creatures. Oh, I understand it, if our physical bodies distress the good senses of the normal world, then imagining us in the act of sex must be a mental toothache. On a deeper level, there is the primal fear that reproduction among or with the disabled would only propagate the worst of the gene pool. I think most people believe only a sick "normal" person would even consider sex with a defective.

Janet is one sick person. Not only did she consider sex with me, she appeared to thoroughly enjoy every aspect of it. She liked it, and she liked it with her eyes wide open and with the lights on. The first time, I was understandably a little self-conscious, but not Janet. She was initiator, facilitator, and in many ways, a competitor. She was also very goal oriented, which became pleasurably apparent when she whispered, "I'm not done with you."

Chapter 2

Lazlow Price carefully prepared the potion in his dimly lit room on Milton Avenue. He could hear the cars whirl past his window, with hurried drivers blasting horns, screeching tires, and gunning engines. Morning rush hour was the loudest, and he welcomed the noise. The noise was good, even when it kept him awake at night. It really didn't matter, because it had been years since Lazlow had slept an entire night. The nightmares always came and brought a quick end to his rest. Images of disgusting creatures filled his nighttime reprieve. God-awful crips, retards and droolers slowly approached him in nightmare after nightmare, trying to sap his strength. They would take and take until there was nothing left, and if he didn't awaken, sweating and fearful, they would take it all, his limbs, his mind, and ultimately his life.

Lazlow really didn't hate them. He really didn't hate mosquitoes, rats, or nighttime barking dogs, either. A well timed slap, mousetrap, or .22-caliber bullet usually eliminated the problem. They were just problems with easy solutions and it was his duty, even his calling in life, to eliminate them. It was also his pleasure. As he used an eye dropper to place the last of the poison in the vial, he knew he was doing God's work, and that thought fortified and energized him. Tomorrow, he would begin the crusade. Tomorrow, Lazlow Price would begin the extermination of human vermin. He would protect normal, God-fearing people, the gene pool, and a society that did not know how to make hard decisions. Today, he would exterminate a life that had no right to live, a life better off dead. As the traffic noise gradually died down, the short, balding, overweight chemistry major with thick, Coke-bottle glasses, continued to concoct a poison that could not easily be detected in a routine autopsy, and that was virtually tasteless. His professors and the Net had taught him well.

Lazlow's part-time day job was completely free from responsibility. He simply poured liquids into bowls, cups and glasses, and plopped meats and fixins onto plates. Five or six hours a day, with two breaks and one lunch hour, he performed this function for hundreds of loud, demanding, hurried students. His co-workers performed the same tasks and rarely spoke to him; their only commonality was the black, spider-web hair nets. The job had been tolerable until the powers-that-be hired one of the disgraces to humanity to perform the identical tasks. She was one of them, and Lazlo knew she must be exterminated.

Chapter 3

It is one of the largest universities in the country. It boasts the most populous dormitory complex and the largest college bus system. There are miles and miles of paved bicycle roads with passing lanes and traffic signs. The university proudly supports three medical schools (human, osteopathic, and veterinary) and a world-famous law school. With strong agricultural roots, it invents new fertilizers, pesticides, and herbicides, and genetically engineers fruits and vegetables. One can even buy "chocolate cheese," somehow obtained from contented campus cows, from a small shop next to the International Center. The International Center is the hub of the campus, located next to the official campus bookstore and housing several specialty stores, dining rooms, coffee shops, and cafes. From it, the library complex can be seen towering over the campus, housing more volumes than any other college in the Midwest. Bell Tower announces the hour and half hour throughout the university and surrounding townships. The campus is lush with trees, grass, bushes, and colorful flowers. The university is a city unto itself. It has its own fire and police departments, preschools, hospitals, and clinics. It dominates the small town that physically surrounds it. Campus and town borders are blurred, and economically, the university is a parasite, drawing apartments, food, and beer from the small, grateful community.

During the fall semester, acres of oak and maple trees brightly color the campus. Fifty thousand students swarm the grounds and buildings, soaking up the rich education they offer. It is a liberal campus, tolerant of everything but intolerance and sometimes freedom of expression. It also serves as a magnet for those students and nonstudents on the fringe of mental stability. On this campus and ones like it, dangerous mental illnesses can be disguised as just another unique way of looking at the world.

The Oak River flows slowly through the southern part of the campus. The public can rent canoes and watch ducks, muskrats, beavers, and turtles do what they have done since the land grant college was legislated into existence. The river winds through the huge groves of trees to a small, unincorporated township where Ma and Pa sell world-class, homemade ice cream. Canoeing upstream is as easy as downstream because the Oak River takes its time, and forces reflection and relaxation on all who venture on it.

Clarene and Donna liked to watch the canoes being launched and captured at the dock. This green spot, next to a huge flowing rose bush, was a favorite lunch hour place for the two day-workers to leisurely eat their homemade sandwiches. On the grassy knoll, high above the dock, they would sit, eat, and take in the beauty the campus had to offer. There was always a comical landing where a canoe would slam into the dock or other canoes, and clumsy, unsure passengers would scramble to the safety of wooden planks. Twice, they had witnessed passengers slip or fall into the muddy river, waist deep in embarrassment. Clarene and Donna never laughed at the wet unfortunates—they were not rude—but they did silently enjoy the lunch hour slapstick nonetheless. Sometimes, back at the apartment, the roommates would recount the events on the Oak River and chuckle, but never meanly. They simply enjoyed seeing normal people, out of their element, stumble, slip and slide when trying to negotiate water and land obstacles. Clarene was always out of her element. Leg braces and cumbersome, primitive crutches helped, but awkwardness was always a part of her life.

Clarene was older than Donna by three years. At twenty-two, she had long ago accepted her physical self. That her spine was deformed at birth was simply a fact of her life. She no longer dreamed of a cure. She was what she was, and that was it. Acceptance had not come easily, but it had come. Clarene was perfectly at ease with herself. Sometimes she even wondered if she would accept a miracle cure if it were offered. She liked herself. Sometimes, when she knew no one would see, she would stare at herself in the full-length mirror in the hall. She was blessed with so many things beautiful. Her long, blond, slightly curly hair ornamented her pleasant facial features and velveteen skin. She wore little makeup, because there was little to make up. She had a typical hourglass frame, at least to her hips. She seldom allowed herself to look below her thin waist at the deformed lower back and legs. She didn't deny their existence; she simply focused on the many positive aspects of her youthful body. Clarene was an optimist.

Donna was a sweet girl. Actually, at nineteen, she was more woman than girl. Down syndrome had given her the physical characteristics once called "Mongoloid." Her round face and slightly slanted eyes made her resemble Chinese Mao more than Nordic Sven, but the oriental reference had long slipped from most people's vocabulary. Down syndrome had restricted Donna to the mental age of a ten-year-old. She did everything like a ten-year-old: reading, writing, speaking and thinking. She was a delightful 10-year-old, but a 10-year-old nonetheless. The only unsettling thing about Donna was that she had the body of a young woman. She was a ten-year-old managing a woman's body.

Janet had negotiated intensely with the reluctant food service company to employ Clarene and Donna. Actually, they hired Clarene on the spot, but needed coaxing, planning and reassurance to hire Donna. Spraying hot water over dirty cups, plates and pots was an ideal job for Clarene. She could sit, spray and then push the tray through the state-of-the-art dish washing machine. Confident legs were not necessary to succeed at this job in the food service industry. But finding a job for Donna was more difficult. Janet had almost given up on gainful employment for the ten-nineteen-year-old when she saw how the plastic spoons, knives and forks had been sorted and carefully wrapped in paper napkins. Instantly, she knew this was a job easily performed by the ten-year-old in the young woman's body. The food service manager finally agreed, and later, similar jobs were added, including stacking clean cups, plates, and pots, which were rinsed by Clarene. To everyone surprise but Janet's, both women were now in their second year of minimum wage employment. The satisfied food service manager even remarked she would be willing to hire more job-hopefuls from the shelter.

"He's kinda scary," confided Clarene, nodding in the direction of the balding, overweight co-worker pouring apple, orange and grapefruit juices into small glasses. Donna glanced in his direction and smiled in agreement. Of course, for Donna, many men were scary, not so much because of their words and actions, but because of the feelings they stirred in her. Very unusual and disquieting feelings. Sometimes, when men stood close to her, she almost tingled with a strange anticipation of something exciting and unknown. She had never told Clarene that the man called "Laz" by the rest of the staff had made her tingle more than most men. The 19-year-old Donna was attracted to the man, but the 10-year-old Donna didn't understand why or where it would lead.

Several times, Donna had approached Laz in an awkward, innocent attempt to spark a deeper relationship, and every time, he had rebuffed her. The rebuffs took many forms, not making eye-contact, walking away mid-sentence or feigning work demands. His seething contempt for her and her kind was not readily apparent to the other workers or to Donna for that matter. Today, however, Laz was uncharacteristically gracious and friendly. During the morning break, both sat together in the employee lounge, apparently enjoying small talk. When Donna went to the restroom, no one saw Laz quickly open her plastic water container, empty the vial of poison in it, tighten the cap, and carefully replace it in her small back pack, next to her brown bag lunch of a ham and cheese sandwich, chips and an apple.

The small family who lived in a rundown married-housing unit had enjoyed the noontime sojourn down Oak River. Robert, a graduate student soon to complete his oral defense of a dissertation exploring a filter's ability to remove *E. coli* bacteria from water, helped his young, pregnant wife and two-year-old son disembark from the narrow, wobbly canoe. As the family of three—soon to be four— finally stood secure on the dock, they heard screams from atop the grassy knoll. Immediately, Robert ran to the aid of the distressed woman, knowing he might be able to help given his training as an EMT, which had paid most of his undergraduate expenses and kept his student loans to a minimum. Reaching the top of the knoll, it was soon apparent that the teenager lying on the grass was in full respiratory arrest. Robert quickly began CPR, which proved to be too little, too late. By the time the ambulance arrived, Donna was dead, although the CPR continued during the ride to the hospital. That sunny midday, Sweet Donna's body was sent to the morgue, and the awful business of informing relatives and friends of a young woman's premature demise began. Janet was the first at the shelter to be given the shocking news.

Chapter 4

Every day Steven Thompson patrolled the campus, he was aware of the lack of respect, the outright disregard students had for the campus police. The students and most of the faculty and staff regarded the campus police as cop "wannabes." They simply did not accept the campus police as "real" cops, a perception that was a thorn in the side of most members of the force. That Steven, and the rest of the campus police department, had the same qualifications as most cops and had completed rigorous training and education programs didn't seem to be general information on this campus with an enrollment larger than many cities. When it came to the real power of the campus police, they carried, and used if necessary, the same pistols and riot control arsenals cops in New York or Los Angeles were issued. Most importantly, the campus police had the same powers to stop, detain and arrest suspects. This campus police department even had a one man detective division, and Steven was it.

Steven was tall, almost too tall for the force. Fortunately, he had missed the maximum height limit by an inch. As the only plainclothes policemen, he was not required to wear a uniform. However, Steven took pride in his appearance, always wore a tie and sport coat, and was ever conscious about the shine on his shoes. His moustache was the only thing in his appearance that was not standard police issue, and it was beginning to show signs of gray. At forty-seven, Steven had been in law enforcement for half of his life. The first years were spent as a military policeman, followed by twelve years with the police department in Laramie, Wyoming. He had been with the campus police more than nine years and was looking forward to completing his career as a campus detective.

Steven had stuttered most of his adult life. In fact, he had stuttered since the third grade. He didn't remember the exact date the stuttering began, or what event caused it; he simply remembered it beginning when he was about eight. The stuttering problem wasn't a severe one. It was barely noticeable most of the time. There were occasions where speech was impossible, but they happened infrequently, and then only when he felt a lot of stress. In the usual incident, Steven just repeated the first sounds of words too many times and occasionally stretched out a word here and there. During severe bouts with the speech disorder, Steven felt his vocal cords close off and stop the air and sounds coming from his mouth. Eventually, the words would come, but only after long, embarrassing, and anxious moments.

The 9-1-1 call from the Oak River boat dock came in about 12:30 p.m. The student wage dispatcher sent the ambulance winding through the crowded campus streets and also notified Steven and the closest cruiser. Steven had just completed the paperwork on two students caught with a marijuana bong in their dorm room. The lab analysis had shown enough residual pot to suspend them from school and require them to attend a drug information program. He knew the Dean of Students wouldn't expel them, and that was fine. After all, it was just pot and carelessness that had resulted in the arrest. A simple slap on the hands was all that was necessary, not that it would do any good in preventing drug abuse by thousands of students. It would simply require them to be more careful about getting caught.

As the senior policeman on campus, Steven got to use the new, white, unmarked sedan recently purchased by the reluctant administration. It was hard to convince the administration, and the faculty law enforcement committee, that the department needed the unmarked car. But after three years of pleading, Steven finally prevailed. When he arrived at the grassy knoll, the ambulance was loading the young woman and futile CPR was being given in earnest. Later, he learned from the intake nurse in the emergency room that the teenager was DOA. He took statements from two students, a married couple who lived on campus and who had been at the dock when the death had occurred. He also interviewed the young woman's roommate, who was picnicking with her. She was in her early twenties and had been understandably upset. Steven was happy to give the handicapped woman a ride to the hospital, and then to her apartment complex.

The dead woman was one of those disabled people one sometimes sees on campus. Most were students, but some worked at menial tasks in dorms or dining rooms. He noted that she had Down syndrome and remembered from some distant conversation that many of the people with this chromosome disorder did not live long lives. Her roommate, Clarene, had informed him that early death was no longer a necessary fate for Down syndrome sufferers. Medical advances prevailed, and many now lived to be parents and even grandparents. However, the medical examiner determined the cause of death to be a heart attack, probably as a result of a preexisting valve irregularity. For Steven, this sad event was opened and closed with little fanfare. People die, and the handicapped are not immune from dying young despite medical advances.

Chapter 5

Janet couldn't believe the news of Donna's death. That such an innocent, pleasant young woman could die so young, so unexpectedly, was a shock to every staff member at the center, especially Janet. But what was even more devastating to Janet was the difficult task of breaking the news to the clients, especially the ones with lower intelligence. For some, the concept of mortality was beyond their reach, for others, the bad news could only be partially understood. Of course, because Janet was the favorite of the clients, the role of bearer of the bad news was her responsibility, one she dreaded.

For the people who only had a passing familiarity with Donna, the news was broken to them in small groups. For the others, the ones who had been her friends, Janet met with them individually. By evening, all of the clients in the shelter knew of Donna's premature demise. That night, Janet went home exhausted, relieved to find the comfort of Ben and bed. He prepared a late dinner, held her quietly, and listened to her into the early morning. They made love and slept the light sleep of mourners, dreading the morning sun, and another day of grief.

Two months later, Lazlow Price worked late into the night, again preparing the death potion. Pleased that his first extermination had been a success, he planned the next act of social cleansing. He knew his job as a food server provided him with unlimited opportunities to dispense death. Since discovering a method of time-release for the poison, another marvelous fact obtained from the Net, Lazlow knew the chances of the police tracing the deaths back to him were remote. Time-released liquids, one of the newest pharmacological miracles, were being used in cough syrup and other liquid medicines, and it was relatively easy for Lazlow to delay the fatal effects of his poison by over an hour.

Lazlow had only seen his next victim a few times. Probably because he had new courses in buildings next to the International Center, the soon-to-be-dead student in a wheelchair had started coming to the cafe for his usual cup of coffee and a bagel. Each time Lazlow saw him in line and served him coffee, he could barely hide his repulsion. Thoroughly disgusted, Lazlow would give him a banana nut bagel and coffee. Today, however, the coffee was more than a beverage. It was a death drug which, in an hour or so, would cleanse the world of yet another despicable creature.

Chapter 6

Although I teach courses in literature, I can't actually say I'm a professor. I only teach one course, and I'm not on that road to happiness known as a tenure-track. Quite frankly, I don't care about tenure or promotion that much. Part time work is just fine with me, and given my latest book royalties, I'm happy just teaching one course a term. I get to teach about a subject I enjoy and get to meet interesting students.

I have a policeman in one of my courses. Actually, he's only a campus cop, but he seems quite competent nonetheless. Over the year, we've become friends. We both look forward to a cup of coffee at the International Center after class where we discuss things related to major British writers. To complete his liberal studies requirements, he is taking my course, and last semester he took my twentieth-century writers course. He's an unusual student, not only because he's older, but his law enforcement experience makes for very interesting discussions.

I wasn't surprised when he told me of the death of the disabled girl. A death on a university campus usually involves a lot of people, and most students and faculty are touched by the rumor mill. When he told me of meeting Janet, and I informed him of our "live in" status, we made the small world comments necessitated by such a coincidence. The world of coincidence got smaller when he told me of the death of another disabled person.

Apparently, a wheelchair bound man also died of a heart attack or something. Steven told me the events surrounding his death. The 30-year-old had been in a motorcycle accident when he was in his teens. His spine was broken, severing the all-important cord which links the brain to the body. He was paralyzed from the waist down and used a state-of-the-art motorized wheelchair to get from place to place. Last year, he enrolled at the university and was seeking a degree in History and Political Science with the goal of taking the Law School Admissions Test and becoming a lawyer. He was going to a morning class on south campus, when his wheelchair plowed into several students. He was hunched over, dead at the controls.

That evening, I told Janet of the demise of yet another disabled person. Although he was not a client at the shelter, she had also heard of his death. We both commented that two deaths occurring in such a short time was unusual.

Chapter 7

Lazlow thought how easy it was to kill them. He doubted the authorities ever thought their deaths were from anything other than natural causes, natural causes for creatures unfit to live in the first place. It was so easy. So clean, and effective. But, the ease of his extermination plan was beginning to bother him, too. There was no lesson for society to learn, and worst of all, no gratitude for a job well done. Early one evening, while the rush hour traffic moaned outside his apartment, Lazlow decided to be more bold, more obvious, and more lethal. He decided to make public his extermination goals. He would not only exterminate an undesirable, he would make a social statement. And to make it public, he would call the student newspaper and announce his intent.

Lazlow both dreaded and was intrigued by the "Major British Writers" liberal studies course he was required to take. He was intrigued by the idea of killing the well-liked professor. As he watched the professor shuffle to the podium, Lazlow silently planned his next extermination. It was one that would undoubtedly bring him national attention and the praise and recognition he deserved. Death would be swift and true, and the campus would buzz with the event within minutes of the deed. Lazlow felt excitement and pride at the act he would perform. He listened to the raspy voice he would silence as the disgusting professor waxed on and on about Chaucer, the writer's perspectives on life and morality, and the filth of the Canterbury Tales. After work, on the walk back to his noisy apartment, Lazlow stopped at a public phone and called the student newspaper. As expected, because it was after hours, he spoke to an answering machine. He calmly read the short, prepared statement from a crumpled sheet of paper he had tucked away in his pocket:

> I am the exterminator of defectives. The world is purer by the death
> of two life forms. The next defective to be exterminated sings the
> praise of a British pornographer. His voice will be silenced. Praise
> be to the Lord.

Lazlow hung up the phone and continued the walk in the cool fall air to his apartment.

The *State News* was run by students, mostly journalism majors. Of course, there was the faculty advisor, Dr. Jennifer Johnson, who served more as a censor than advisor. When Professor Johnson heard the recording of the exterminator's threat, she knew it shouldn't be taken lightly. The *State News* had run both stories of the deaths of the disabled people and she remembered them clearly. Both articles stated their deaths were the result of natural causes. Now, the advisor was not certain. After the excited student who had brought her the answering machine recording left, she called campus police.

After meeting with Professor Johnson, Steven Thompson called the Federal Bureau of Investigation and spoke to an impatient receptionist who had little tolerance for his stutter. Treating him as if he were retarded, she finally connected him to the appropriate special agent for the region. Steve wondered how special an agent was if every agent in the Bureau was called "special." By the next day, the small campus police headquarters was crowded with clean-cut, suit-wearing F.B.I. agents, "fibies" as they were called in Wyoming, trained to deal with homicides and death threats. Within hours of their arrival, a judge had ordered exhumation of Donna's and the pre-law student's bodies. The extensive autopsies conducted by the F.B.I. pathologist found traces of the poison which had resulted in their deaths. On the death certificates, demise from "natural causes" was now changed to "homicide." The murder investigations began in earnest.

Chapter 8

After reading the *State News* article about the death threat, I began to feel uneasy. In the recesses of my mind, I entertained the idea that I might be next on the hit man's list. I was certainly a candidate. I was disabled, on campus, and highly visible. At dinner that evening, Janet also noted that many students consider some of the Canterbury Tales sexually explicit, and some might even consider them pornography. Was it a coincidence that in the past week my lectures were about Chaucer?

Initially, Steven downplayed my concerns, but as we talked about motives and opportunities, he too began to suspect I might be next. The following day we met in my office, and went over the list of students in my Major British Writers course. I had one section of the course with a total enrollment of more than 150. Steven methodologically scanned the enrollment roster for names of students with any criminal history. Two students were found to have a rap sheet, but both offenses were for "driving under the influence." A third student had been arrested for shoplifting in her freshman year. All three students were eliminated as possible suspects. By afternoon, we both accepted the fact that I was vulnerable and that my fears were real. Steven said I should seriously consider canceling my course, and remaining in my apartment or leaving town until the murderer was apprehended. The minute he made the suggestions that I run and hide from harm's way, I knew it would never happen.

I'm simply not the kind of person to run from a threat. Maybe it's because of my disabilities. I have never been able to run from them, either. They're real and ever present. In my experience you confront and deal with them, or forever run. And the running is not really from them, it is from your self, and there is no place to hide. I have embraced all that is me: the good, the bad, and the ugly. We don't live in a perfect world, and there are few of us who even approach perfection. As Popeye so philosophically noted, "I yam what I yam, and that's all I yam." Well, if there was a crazed killer out there determined to eliminate me, then so be it. I would do what I could to prevent it. Hell, I would do everything I could to keep living, but I wouldn't run and hide. It was not in my constitution. I just wouldn't do it.

Steven and I listened to the recording with the terse threat on it, hoping I might be able to recognize the voice. But with over 150 students, it was futile, mostly because I have never met the majority of my students, let alone had a conversation with them. My class is a standard lecture one, "a sage on stage," as some call it. Occasionally, a student will ask a question or offer a comment, but even that is a rare occurrence. The course is held three times a week, with each lecture lasting fifty minutes. It's not an interactive course; there is very little student participation.

In my first novel, *Murder in Montana*, I had done some research on speech recognition devices. The plot of the novel revolved around a corporate employee who had stolen and sold the formula for a powerful antidote to several lethal gases that were used in the Gulf War. He had then changed his identity, and with the profits from selling the secrets of the antidote, moved to West Yellowstone, Montana to enjoy the spoils of his crime. During research for the book, I discovered many high-tech companies were using two types of identification systems to allow selective access to secret computer files. A widely used authorization device is a retina scan. Laser light scans a person's retina, and because no two are identical, positive identification can be made. Once the domain of science fiction, retina scanning has now become relatively commonplace in high-tech companies and governmental agencies.

The second type of identification is through voice prints. As with retinas, no two individuals' voice and speech patterns are identical. Voice prints are more useful than retina scans because most computers, even laptops, have embedded microphones which permit this type of speaker recognition. All a person has to do is to speak a series of words, which have been previously analyzed, into the microphone, and the computer then either denies or allows access to documents and data based on the acoustical analysis. In my novel, access to the antidote formula was permitted using this type of device.

Steven and I were convinced that the murderer was a member of my Major British Writers course. First, he had used the word "defectives." In my courses, I sometimes jokingly refer to myself as a defective when I drop lecture notes or chalk, or have to repeat myself due to my speech disorder. I say something like, "Pardon my defective speech," or "It's not easy being a defective." These comments usually bring lighthearted laughter to the classroom and make the students feel more at ease with me and my disabilities. Second, the murderer made the pornography comment, this occurring during my lectures on Chaucer. Granted, all of this is circumstantial evidence at best, but at least it was something. Steven and I agreed if we could somehow get a voice sample from each student, we could compare them to the answering machine recording. The big problem was how to obtain a speech sample with one or more of the words used on the threatening recording. For accurate analysis, the same word has to be used for comparison purposes.

Steven and I carefully analyzed the transcript of the answering machine recording. How could I get all 150 students to say one or more of the words on the recording? *I am the exterminator of defectives. The world is purer by the death of two life forms. The next defective to be exterminated sings the praise of a British pornographer. His voice will be silenced. Praise be to the Lord.* My first thought was the word "I." It is the most frequently used word in English. But, how to get the students to say it? Steven and I sat stooped over the sample for hours until in frustration we decided to sleep on it. After all, I had to prepare the midterm examination.

Sometimes in my sleep I solve problems. I understand this is not necessarily unusual. Many people wake up with a solution to a nagging problem. I have heard that Einstein solved a major mathematical problem in his sleep. Somehow, during sleep, the mind is free to explore options or to allow solutions to surface. And maybe, because I'm disabled, the freedom of dreaming is more important in problem-solving. That morning at precisely 4:30, it hit me. I woke Janet and told her of the solution, as much to share the revelation as to ensure that I would not go back to sleep and forget it.

As soon as Steven got to his office, I called and told him of my plan. I would get a speech sample from all of the students during the examination. I also resolved to keep my investigation from the F.B.I. I doubted my plan would be constitutional.

When Lazlow Price read the small *State News* article about the death threat, he became furious. It was just a small article, hidden on page nine of the paper. Worst of all, no local television or newspapers picked it up. What infuriated Lazlow more than anything was that they didn't take him seriously. Apparently to them he was just another crackpot. Well, he resolved, they'll be taught a lesson and soon.

Chapter 9

The Department of Speech and Hearing Sciences is located on the third floor of Building 6 of the Health Sciences Complex. Steven and I made an appointment to meet with one of the professors knowledgeable about voice prints. Dr. Oscar Sciacca, a senior faculty member and specialist in the acoustics of speech, expressed immediate interest in our situation, and said he could compare the voice prints of the 150 students. He would use two research assistants to help with the tedious aspects of preparing the voice samples. As we walked with him to his laboratory, he asked the whys, whats and wherefores about the project. Steven provided him with detailed information about the death threat and how we intended to get the voice samples. Dr. Sciacca suggested we get the actual telephone and answering machine from the *State News* office because he would need them to do the analysis of the speech samples. Apparently, telephones and audio recorders vary in their frequency responses. He also wanted the audio recorder we would be using to obtain the speech samples from the students.

Examination day is stressful for everyone—students, teaching assistants, and professors alike. Today was no exception, especially since I suspected one of my students was planning to murder me. Once the students had filed into my classroom, I had my two teaching assistants distribute the computer grading sheets to them. As soon as they settled down, I briefly welcomed them to the class, and asked that they fill in the blanks and darken the small dots indicating their name, seat and social security numbers. While they were busily working their number two pencils, I casually took three photographs of the classroom with my small, old camera.

After the doors were closed and locked, my teaching assistants began distributing the examination. The students believed there were several forms of this examination and they, upon receiving the exam, needed to tell the teaching assistants which one they had. Prior to distributing the exam, I had written the words "Form Two" at the top of first page of every test. I told the students that because of computer problems, they must tell the teaching assistants their names and which form they received. Because I wanted them to have the full fifty minutes to finish the exam, they would speak their names and form numbers into a small digital audio recorder held about six inches from their lips. The teaching assistant would then have a record of the student's name and form number to ensure proper grading of the exams. I apologized for the computer glitch, but assured them that it was necessary if grading was to be accurate. I made up a phony story about the problems the Central Scanning Department was having with their new hardware. As the students received their tests, each one spoke his or her name and the same words, "Form Two," into the audio recorder held by the teaching assistants.

No student questioned the change in testing protocol and this didn't surprise me. The students were simply too preoccupied with remembering the information, completing the exam, and getting home for much needed sleep after hours of cramming. The collecting of speech samples was completed without a hitch. Three students had left messages on my voice mail indicating they could not take the examination at the designated time because of family emergencies or illnesses. Fortunately, all three were female, and we excluded them from the suspect list.

Steven was waiting for me at my office when I returned after the last test had been completed by the slowest student. I thought it was overkill and a little dramatic, but Steven used the siren and flashing portable light of his car to get us to Dr. Sciacca's lab. He and his two assistants were analyzing the speech samples within fifteen minutes of our arrival. Steven waited at the speech acoustics lab while I took the film to be developed. I knew there was a photo shop in the International Center. I called Janet from my cell phone as I walked past the libraries. She agreed to meet with me, and have a cup of decaffeinated latte at "our" coffee shop in the International Center. We frequently met there after my class. It was sort of a pleasant ritual begun years ago when we first started dating.

Steven offered to help Dr. Sciacca and the lab assistants. They politely refused his help and he silently wondered if it was because of his stutter. During the past week or so, it had been getting worse, probably a result of the stress he was feeling about the murders and danger Ben was in. He always admired Ben for his intellect. He was one of the most intelligent people he'd ever met. Now, he also admired him for his courage. Steven saw him differently since he'd refused to stay home or leave the campus until the murderer was caught. He knew Ben was afraid, but he wasn't about to let some crackpot make him run and hide. He wouldn't buckle. Steven knew Ben saw the murderer much like he viewed his own disabilities. Ben confronted these trials and tribulations much like he did his cerebral palsy—straight ahead. Ben was a courageous man.

A voice print breaks the speech signal into three components: time, frequency and energy. The computer readout, called a spectrogram, shows small, detailed aspects about these three components. Although all words have basic similarities in time, frequency and energy, there are minor individual variations among different speakers. One way of looking at it is that a person's head is a resonating chamber, much like a musical instrument such as a violin or trombone. The vocal cords serve as a source of vibration, and certain aspects of that energy are amplified or damped by a person's head. Because people's heads, or resonating chambers, are different, their spectrograms are different. Even identical twins have different spectrograms because, although their heads are identical, they have learned to speak differently. For example, one twin might produce the /s/ sound a little longer in duration than the other twin. These differences are in milliseconds. Also, there might be small differences between the length of pauses between sounds, the way voice onset occurs, or how the pitch rises at the end of a vowel in anticipation of another sound. These are a result of individual learning, and no two people share all of them. There are many other little variations that can be detected. Voice print analysis consists of looking at these resonance and speech pattern differences for consistency. In the past, the analysis took days, even weeks, but now they are rapidly and accurately done by computers.

About an hour after the voice analyses began, Dr. Sciacca and his assistants made a positive match. Speech sample eleven, a male by the name of Lazlow Price, had a 95% positive match with the word "Form" and a 97% accuracy value with the word "Two." Steven immediately logged onto the police department's computer and searched the records for a Mr. Lazlow Price. He found no wants or warrants, and no significant rap sheet other than three parking violations. He then searched the administration records and found the suspect had several student loans and part-time employment at one of the cafes in the International Center. In fact, it was a coffee shop frequented by Ben who was probably there now waiting for the film to be developed. Ben had a weakness for decaffeinated latte. Suddenly, Steven feared for his friend's life.

As Steven rushed to his car, he tried several times to call Ben on his cell phone. There was no answer. Ben must have forgotten to turn it on. As he sped through the narrow campus streets with siren blasting and light flashing, he had the dispatcher send a cruiser to the coffee shop. He doubted the cruiser would beat him there, but this was one of those situations where time definitely was of the essence.

Janet was already at a table sipping her coffee. Actually, she was sipping the whipped cream generously plopped atop it. I ordered my usual from one of the familiar faces doing the serving and soon was sitting next to my beautiful girlfriend. In the distance, I could hear the "wherrrr" of a siren and assumed another pedestrian had been clipped at an intersection, a frequent and unfortunate occurrence on this busy campus. As I reached for my first sip of coffee, my spastic muscles caused an overshooting of movement, and I spilled some of the hot beverage on my lap, not exactly an unusual occurrence for me. I told Janet my muscles were clumsier today, probably because of the cold, autumn wind. I wiped it off using a paper napkin, which had been wrapped around plastic eating utensils, and began to clean my slacks when I saw Steven's car screech to a stop. He ran to our table and stutteringly asked if I'd drunk or eaten anything. He ordered the other officers, who had just arrived, to secure the place for evidence, hurried us into his car, and sped to the safety of the campus police department.

It's been seven weeks since my brush with death. I find it ironic that my clumsy spastic muscles actually saved my life by delaying my first sip of coffee. The F.B.I. lab analysis showed a high amount of poison, which would have certainly caused my heart to seize. The campus cops arrested Lazlow Price at the scene and charged him with two cases of murder in the first degree and one case of attempting to murder me. He is now in jail, being held there without bond. Janet had been right from the beginning. Sometimes, just sometimes, being disabled in a blessing in disguise.

"Murphy's Inner World of Aphasia" was originally published in *The Family Guide to Surviving Stroke and Communication Disorders* (Pearson Allyn & Bacon Publishers) and *The Family Guide to Surviving Stroke and Communication Disorders* (2nd edition) (Jones and Bartlett Publishers).

He liked to be called "Murph," which was short for Murphy. Three years into retirement, he and Beth, his wife of forty-five years, were well adjusted to the leisure life. Well, it was not exactly a life of leisure; the chores continued. Some days, it seemed retirement was more demanding and more active than the workaday world. To Murph, if retirement was not the life of leisure he had always dreamed it would be, at least he set his own pace. And that meant a lot. Today was to be a typical day in the world of the retired, and it was typical, except for one thing. In the next few hours, Murph's life would change forever. Murph would have a stroke.

The Great Cross-Country Journey was scheduled to begin next week. The pre-owned Bounder motor home had set them back a pretty penny. But what a great machine: two televisions, a microwave, a DVD player, and plenty of storage. Murphy would have preferred a diesel rather than gas engine, but gas was relatively cheap. At seven miles to the gallon, it needed to be.

They had owned the machine two weeks and Murph did not have buyer's remorse. In fact, he had buyer's glee over the best looking recreational vehicle he'd ever seen, let alone owned. The Bounder made Murph happier than he'd been in years. When Beth was out shopping, he climbed up into the driver's seat and just sat. Murph felt like he was on top of the world. He knew what people said about men and boys and the price of their toys. He also didn't care.

Murph knew he had a lot to do before embarking on the great adventure. The Bounder was in good shape but needed some TLC to be brought up to his high standards. Murph had always been a perfectionist. His son, Matt, offered to help with the preparations, but Murph didn't like to impose on anyone, especially Matt. He knew Matt's twins were a handful, and his free time was limited, what with overtime and all. The birth of the twins had stretched Matt's finances to the limit. Matt's wife, Andrea, had to return to work much too soon after the birth of Murph and Beth's only grandchildren. Murph felt a pang of guilt about spending so much money on the Bounder, but as they say in beer commercials, "You only go around once."

As Murph got into his pickup to go to the auto-parts store to buy road flares he hoped they would never need, a twinge of tightness gripped his right arm. For a moment, he could not open the door. The aging pickup always had a sticky door, but this seemed unusual. "Oh well," he thought to himself, "I'll buy some oil for the hinges when I get to the store."

Driving to the store, Murphy tuned in to his favorite radio station. "The Country Voice of the Valley," they liked to proclaim. The nasal country tunes and the late morning sunshine made his increasing anxiety about the tightness in his arm dissolve. He had always liked country music; it was honest and all that. He couldn't imagine listening to anything else. As Murph pulled into the auto-parts store, he hit the curb with too much force. The jolt was enough to test the strength of the seat belt.

"Damn," he thought, "There goes the front-end alignment. Now I'll have to get...to get...What's that called..."

Murphy stepped out of the pickup and started walking to the entrance of the store. As he opened the door, again his right arm wouldn't do as he wanted. He stood there for a minute in confusion.

"What's wrong with my arm?" he asked no one in particular.

On the way home, Murph was again at peace with the world. The guilt pangs about spending too much money on the Bounder still nudged at his conscience, but the confusion and anxiety slipped away. "Ah, the curative effects of country music," he thought.

Murph had always been one to ignore fear. He realized during the war he had been more lucky than invincible and more lonely than fearful. Like most of his generation, the war made him realize a lot. Whenever fear reared its ugly head, he was able to kick it back where it belonged. This method of coping worked well throughout his life. Murph had the gift of "If it bothers you, ignore it; it'll go away."

When Murphy got home, Beth was gone, probably visiting Matt, Andrea, and the twins. He didn't mind. He'd make one of his world class sandwiches for lunch. Today, the sandwich would consist of three slices of ham, Swiss cheese, a dollop of horseradish sauce, a pickle, and a tad of mustard. There was no wheat bread, so he settled for the last two slices of white. Had Beth been home, she would have objected to the sandwich. She spent way too much time worrying about blood pressure, cholesterol, and salt intake. The sandwich was delicious and as the last bite was swallowed, Beth walked through the door. That afternoon, Murph mentioned the problems with his arm and hand. He managed to work it into the conversation while complaining about his usual aches and pains. He minimized the event more to protect himself from the disturbing thoughts than to prevent her from overreacting.

Murph and Beth spent an uneventful evening together. After dinner, they talked about little things. She pretended to be interested in the playoffs, and he listened to more concerns about the grandchildren. There was a comfortable routine to their lives. It wasn't exciting, but it was predictable and secure. After the television was turned off, they retired to the bedroom. Murph's last words to Beth were, "Did you lock the doors?" As usual, he was asleep within minutes of his head hitting the pillow.

Murph was an early riser. It was hard for him to sleep with the sun up. He considered himself a hard worker. Hard workers get up early, work hard, and go to bed tired. At 5:30 a.m., Murph opened his eyes. He felt the warm, comforting presence of Beth next to him. He heard her soft snore—well, not a snore exactly, more of a muffled buzz. Beth was quite adamant about the fact that ladies do not snore. He quietly got up, always careful not to awaken his mate. If Murph was an early riser, Beth was the consummate night owl. A lark married to an owl. Of course, Murph needed and always received a little catnap during the day. It was one of the perks of retirement. He silently planned the day's activities, careful to schedule that all important catnap. His biggest concern was a problem with the Bounder's air conditioning. "This could be an expensive day," he thought to himself.

As Murph walked toward the bathroom, he felt the strange sensation in his right arm again. His first reaction was one of irritation. He didn't have time for this nonsense. Only this time, it was not limited to his arm; the whole right side of his body felt strange. Suddenly, for the first time in a long time, Murphy was afraid. As he reached the bathroom door, his right side gave way and he tumbled into the dresser. He tried to catch himself, but to no avail. The family pictures carefully aligned on the dresser crashed to the floor, causing Beth to awaken and ask, "What's wrong, Murph?"

Murph didn't answer. He didn't understand the question. "Who's on?" he thought. What a strange thing for her to say.

Murph tried to get up, but it was no use. The entire right side of his body would not budge. Try as he would, Murph could not make his body move. Not his leg, arm, or hand. "This can't be happening," he thought.

"What a strange dream," was his last coherent thought. Murph lost consciousness.

Beth was awakened by the startling early morning noise. Why would Murph knock the family pictures to the floor? It took only an instant for Beth to register the events completely: Murphy was having a stroke. Maybe he was dying. She should have seen it coming. Strangely, Beth's immediate concern was the pictures on the floor and the broken glass. "Someone could get cut," she thought. Then she had the presence of mind to ask Murphy, "What's wrong?" There was no reply.

Beth dialed 9-1-1 on the bedroom telephone. "Nine, one, one. What's your emergency?" was the matter-of-fact voice on the other end. Within 20 minutes, 20 long minutes, the paramedics arrived. The flashing lights woke the neighbors. There were sounds of police and ambulance radios, and a stretcher was brought to the bedroom.

"It's clear the shush is," Murphy slurred.

"He's delirious," thought Beth. She knelt down and tried to comfort him.

Murph kept saying the strangest things. "It's shush, beyond." The utterances turned into unintelligible sounds and finally silence as Murphy gradually slipped into unconsciousness. Beth couldn't get the image of Murph lying on the bedroom floor out of her mind. It seemed so odd.

Beth saw the ambulance rush Murph off to the hospital. She was sure this was just a minor and temporary problem. No way could this be happening to her. Murphy was too strong to fall victim to something like this. A feeling of calm surrounded her as she got into the car to drive to the hospital. There was relief in blotting from her mind the terrible things that were happening to her and Murphy.

Apparently, one of the neighbors called Matt and Andrea. They met Beth at the hospital's main waiting room. It was good to see familiar faces. They hugged and talked grimly in low voices about the early morning shock. Beth was on the verge of tears. It was hard for her to stay in control; she was afraid of what this day would bring.

Murphy was brought into the emergency room. He became aware of the hustle and bustle, and it frightened him. It was too intense, too hectic. He was placed on heart, oxygen, and blood pressure monitors. Blood was taken for the lab tests, and oxygen tubes were placed in his nose. He was awake during most of the chaotic activities but had little understanding of what was happening. It was like a movie, a bad movie. A catheter was inserted to help with urination.

Twice, Murphy asked for Beth. Unfortunately, to the triage nurse it sounded like, "Care for mother." Murphy couldn't understand why the nurses, technicians, and doctors didn't seem to understand his perfectly normal speech. He drifted into the sanctuary of sleep. Later that morning, Murphy had a vague sensation of claustrophobia while the CT (computerized axial tomography) brain scan was conducted. He wanted to express his fear, but was too tired to do so. He did not like being slid into the small tube. One thing bothered Murphy more than the claustrophobia—the shouting. Everyone felt the need to shout instructions. They moved their heads close to his ear and shouted things Murphy was incapable of understanding. Apparently, they felt Murphy had lost his hearing.

Dr. William Tobbler, a board-certified neurologist, was on call all night. It had been a long night. He evaluated a youngster with a severe head injury. Seizure after seizure shook the little fellow's body. The seizures were finally under control, at least for now. As he watched the elderly man being wheeled into intensive care, he wondered if his services would be required. The man was pale, obviously paralyzed on the right side, and he heard the nurse say he couldn't communicate; he was aphasic.

He saw the hospital's oldest staff physician, John Foster, trailing after the new patient. John had his usual sour look and permanent frown plastered on his face. He liked Foster and the old-fashioned "country doctor" role he played. Watching him was like watching a rerun of Marcus Welby, M.D. John was considered a medical jack-of-all-trades.

The intensive care unit (ICU) is a strange place. Technology rules supreme and the patients, the ones with the illnesses and injuries, appear to be an afterthought. The incessant beeping, clicking, and humming of the expensive machines are constant companions to staff and patients alike. In this hospital, there were 12 intensive care rooms. Murphy was placed in ICU-3. He lay on his back, a stiff sheet covering his body and the multitude of tubes and cords leading to and from him. The curtains were drawn, and the mute images of television flashed in the dimly lit room. Murphy drifted in and out of sleep during most of the hours spent in the emergency room. He felt like an observer of the strange events occurring to him. It was easier to be an observer than a participant because it was all so unreal.

The first permanent memory Murph had of the ICU was the odor: disinfectant. There was no question in his mind that he was in a hospital; nothing smelled as clean and sterile as alcohol, and hospitals are drenched in it. Murph looked around. He recognized a few of the machines and most of the room's objects. He noted the tubes and lines attached to his body, and felt the irritation of patches securing the sensors to his chest and arm. His mouth was dry and felt like it had cotton stuffed inside. The oxygen tubes in his nose bothered him; he wanted to pull them out. Suddenly, panic gripped him; his hands were tied to the bed. He struggled, but it was no use. In hospital terminology, he was restrained, and restrained well. He couldn't scratch an itch if his life depended on it.

As Murph lay back, succumbing to the restraints, he felt calm; a sense of well-being surrounded him. As he stared at the hospital ceiling, he simply denied what had happened. He convinced himself nothing bad was happening and if it was, it wasn't happening to him. He welcomed the break from reality, and he slipped into the sanctuary of sleep.

When he awoke, Murph sensed he was in trouble. Something bad had happened. Hospital rooms like this were for people on the verge of death. From deep within his mind, thoughts of escaping from this dangerous place welled up. But strangely, he had no words to carry the thoughts. The only thing present was the overwhelming need to escape. "Get me out of here!" was vocalized as nothing. No words came to his mind and no movements came to his lips. If Murph could have talked, he would have shouted: "I can't talk, help me!"

Beth met with Dr. Foster in the coffee shop. "It's serious, Beth," Dr. Foster pronounced. "He's had a serious stroke and he might not make it. Even if he does pull through his speech and ability to walk have been affected."

This declaration was no surprise to Beth. She knew it was bad and Dr. Foster only confirmed it. A wave of sadness washed over her. It was the kind of feeling you get when a loved one is in serious trouble. Her first thought was to share this sad feeling with Murph. He'd understand the depth of it. He'd be strong.

Many doctors would have said to this anxious woman, "The CT scan showed an infarct in the left frontal region of the cortex without a midline shift." Not Dr. John Foster. He decided a long time ago that this type of medico-jargon was a form of verbal abuse. He would never talk to family members, and especially his old friend Beth, like that. He simply said, "The X-ray showed damage on the left side of the brain where speech is found. It is also the area that controls the right arm and leg. In fact, in Murph's case, the entire right side of his body may be paralyzed. It appears to be a clot and not a broken blood vessel."

Dr. Foster took the time to explain as much as he could to Beth.

"Yes, it's early."

"No, he's asleep now."

"Yes, his heart is strong."

"Yes, the stroke could get worse."

"No, brain cells do not grow back."

"No, he's not in a coma."

"Yes, he'll recognize you."

"No, he's not in physical pain."

"Our first goal is to get him stabilized, and then we'll begin thinking about rehabilitation," Dr. Foster planned aloud. He wanted to go into more detail but heard the blare of his telephone. He checked the number and politely ended the conversation. As he walked off, Beth felt angry as the realities of the situation set in. She was angry with Dr. Foster for confirming the bad news, and mad at herself for not doing something to prevent the stroke. She was also mad at Murphy for not taking better care of himself. All she could think was, "Why did this have to happen?" Beth was left alone in the crowded room, more alone than she had ever been.

Back in ICU, Murph saw Beth, Matt, and Andrea enter the room. Their grim faces triggered another bout of anxiety. He imagined their sad faces at his funeral. "Where are the twins?" he wondered in wordless thought. Their young, identical faces always brought a smile. Murph did not like the sad, forlorn faces on the three people he loved. He tried to say that it was all right and that things were going to be just fine, but there were no words, no sounds, no nothing. All that was present were images and sensations; there was no language to bring order to thought. He heard one and only one word surface to his mind's ear: "Weird." As he attempted to verbalize it, nothing happened. As he tried again and again to express the weirdness of it all, his lips, tongue, and voice box suppressed it. The harder he tried, and the more force he brought to bear, the harder it was to command the movements of speech. With every increased effort to say, "W—eer—d," there was a corresponding increase in the resistance to program it. There were so few words he could remember, and when they did come to mind, they were too complicated to utter. Weird indeed.

Beth was careful not to disrupt the IV needle when she took Murph's hand. Her warm, firm hand in his was the first pleasant, comforting sensation Murph experienced since his swan dive into the dresser. Tears swelled in his eyes and uncontrollable sobbing followed. Murph found himself crying like a baby. The crying was way out of proportion to the feelings he was experiencing. He wasn't that emotional or that sad. Talk about embarrassing. The nurse observing the family meeting made a mental note that Murphy was "emotionally labile." She heard the doctors use those terms to indicate a patient who has exaggerated emotions due to brain damage.

Matt and Andrea were at a loss for words. They made small talk about the twins and other things, but it didn't take long for them to realize that the conversation was one sided. Murph saw tears in Andrea's eyes, and once again he cried. The embarrassment he felt was incredible. He tried to explain, but once again, all that came out was blathering nonsense. Murph never felt so out of control, so utterly helpless. On a nonverbal level, he knew if this was to be his future, death would be a welcome event.

As chance would have it, Dr. Tobbler arrived to consult on the patient in ICU-3 when Beth, Matt, and Andrea were there. He shook hands with the family and began to explain the medications Murphy was taking. The results of the CT scan were explained in frightening detail. Apparently, Murph was scheduled for an MRI—magnetic resonance imagery—to further help pinpoint the site of the brain damage. Dr. Tobbler said Murph's stroke was no longer in evolution, which Beth deduced was a good thing. It wouldn't get worse. In a day or two, Murph would be transferred to a regular hospital room.

Day two for Murph was as bad as day one. In fact, it was worse. The lunch tray was placed in front of him, and the nurse helped make the food manageable for a man with movement only on his left side. It was a puree diet, one obviously meant for stroke patients. Murph could barely manage the movement of the spoon to his mouth with his left hand, so a nurse's aide was sent in to help him. He knew the reputation of hospital food but it did taste good. In fact, the smell, texture, and taste were welcome, familiar sensations. The nurse's aide was careful to keep the gray, brown, and yellow spoonfuls confined to the general area of his mouth. More embarrassment and more blows to his self-esteem. Murph had an image of himself as an ugly, overgrown baby with food smeared all over his mouth. But the real embarrassment was yet to come.

During the night, Murph's bowels moved. He felt the sensations and tried to call for the nurse but was unsuccessful. He knew he needed to call for a bedpan or to get up and go to the bathroom, but he didn't have the words to plan the acts. He wasn't confused; he knew what was going on. He was perplexed, and couldn't organize himself well enough to push the call light. He couldn't remember how to shout for the nurse.

He lay in his own waste, the smell overwhelming. On the most basic of levels, Murphy knew this was absolutely the worst thing that had ever happened to him. A kind nurse's aide came to his rescue. She cleaned him and the mess. Murph watched her face carefully for any indication of scorn or ridicule. None was detected and Murph was glad for that. There were few things to be glad about. As she prepared to leave, Murph tried to utter something, anything, to lessen the embarrassment. Of course, even if he had been the most eloquent speaker in the world, nothing would have eased the awkwardness. Murph had the lowest image of himself he ever had. The stroke turned him into a babbling, drooling child, lying in his own waste. A little later, Beth entered the room and quietly sat down.

More words were becoming available to Murph. Fragments of complete inner statements occasionally came to mind. However, his verbal thoughts and visual imagery rarely connected. Occasionally he understood the words of others. He had the most difficulty when people spoke rapidly or strung long sentences together. Dr. Foster asked him if he felt pain, and Murphy was convinced the good doctor was informing him of the needed rain. Beth brought in a pencil and paper, hoping Murph could write his thoughts. Another blow to Murph's self-esteem: he wrote like a child. All he could muster were scribbles and a few lines resembling his name. Everyone who saw the scribbles thought he was writing something profound. Matt saw the Bounder, Andrea saw the twins, and one nurse hurriedly brought him a bedpan. His writing was a makeshift inkblot test.

Dr. Linda Curzon was a 34-year-old physiatrist. She had been out of medical school only a few years, but was more certain than ever that physical medicine and rehabilitation was the right specialty for her. She knew her trade and knew it well. The consult on the stroke patient in ICU-3 came early in the day. The attending physician was Dr. Foster. She'd had problems with Dr. Foster in the past. Old docs often tried to be one-man shows and resisted seeking her, or any other specialist's, opinion. She was director of rehabilitation and vice president of the medical staff, and it might be that Dr. Foster was resentful of her age or specialty. That was his problem. She was a busy woman. She performed her usual thorough evaluation for rehabilitation potential on Murphy. There was a gleam in his eyes that she liked. The spark of life was still there.

During the course of her examination, Dr. Curzon became angry. A tray was ordered for this patient and the nurses eagerly fed the poor fellow. His face sagged, his tongue deviated on protrusion, his vocal cords would not close completely, and the gag reflex was absent. A first-year intern would have known he was at risk for aspiration pneumonia. His temperature had spiked, and a person had to be deaf not to hear the gurgle in his lungs. Murph was sick and getting sicker. She placed him on NPO (nothing orally) status and ordered a chest X-ray along with a speech and swallowing evaluation. She also ordered physical and occupational therapy. Her most pressing concerns were the swallowing problems and potential for aspiration pneumonia.

Wendy, a certified speech-language pathologist, loved her interactions with the patients, but hated the paperwork. The almighty paperwork. It wasn't even paperwork anymore, because the hospital had been computerized. All notes were entered into the central computer and one had to request a printout to even see paperwork.

Documentation, documentation, and more documentation. Sometimes she felt she spent more time satisfying needs of the bureaucrats and HMO's than the needs of the patients. As Wendy walked out of the therapy suite, the secretary pulled a slip of paper from her mailbox. Apparently, there was a new speech evaluation in ICU-3. A stroke patient of Dr. Foster's with aspiration pneumonia.

When Wendy walked into the ICU, she saw a nurse's aide leave the patient's room. The lingering odor spoke volumes of what had just happened. "The poor guy," Wendy thought. She said "Hello" to one of the familiar faces in the unit and received a forced obligatory nod. "They ought to rename this the insensitive care unit," Wendy thought as she typed her personal identification code into the unit's computer. Quickly, a complete history of the medical life and times of the patient was made available. She read his history, procedures, and consults with care. "Rather young to be losing so much," she thought. In her business, young was relative.

She walked into Murph's room and surveyed the situation. The woman sitting next to the bed was probably his wife, but Wendy learned a long time ago not to make assumptions about relationships. Murph had his eyes closed, but she suspected he was not asleep. Many patients kept their eyes closed, especially after embarrassing events. It was a basic method of escape and avoidance. Gray, thinning hair, thick eyebrows, and a bit on the heavy side; Murph was definitely the grandfather type.

Wendy greeted the woman seated next to the bed. She offered the details expected of her by providing her name and profession. She explained that her job was to evaluate

Murph's speech, voice, language, and swallowing abilities. When that was completed, she would provide therapy to help the patient recover as much as possible. Beth heard the same kind of speech from the physical and occupational therapists; only the names and faces changed. Wendy was careful to project both professionalism and empathy in the first contact. The negativity often associated with strokes could interfere with the working relationship if the clinician was not careful.

"Good afternoon" were the first words Wendy said to Murph. He opened his eyes and saw a young woman standing by his bed. He recognized the two words as a greeting but didn't know if she was bidding him good morning, good day, or good night. He smiled and nodded his head. Murph had already been stung too often with the pain of verbal impotence to attempt speech. Murph learned quickly that it was a verbal crapshoot every time he opened his mouth. Occasionally, he said the correct word, but more often than not, nothing came out or he blurted out the unexpected. Murphy sensed this woman was responsible not for his blood, urine, walking, dressing, or breathing; she was here for his speech. He felt his first vague sense of hope.

Each time Murph tried to talk to Wendy, he fought to remember the word or struggled to program it. Even when he remembered the word and programmed it into existence, he produced it with a slur, a distortion caused by weak speech muscles. So far, all of his speech had been whispered. The familiar buzz of his voice box was absent. As Wendy tested his understanding of words, ability to sequence strings of sounds and syllables, and strength of speech muscles, Murph did his best to comply. After all, Murph had always been a hard worker and prided himself on that fact. Murph was glad someone in the hospital understood the problems he was having with his speech. Wendy really understood. He could tell. She had seen other people adrift in this verbal confusion. Then Murph had another realization: he was not the only person who had ever had this problem. Wendy finished her evaluation and talked to Beth about him. Beth nodded her head and asked questions. Occasionally, they both looked in Murph's direction.

Murph felt like a visitor in a strange, technologically advanced country. He didn't speak or understand the language of these foreigners. He recognized the objects, utensils, pictures, and uniforms as objects, utensils, pictures, and uniforms. The problem was that the names were different, or completely absent, in this strange foreign country. Most unusual.

The next morning, Murph was lifted from his bed to a wheelchair. He tried to help with the transfer but found he was dead weight. So many times in his life he had gotten out of bed and so often he had taken it for granted. He would never take easy movement for granted again.

As he was wheeled to the radiology section of the hospital, the people he passed in the halls and elevator greeted him in an uneasy manner. All he could do was nod his head and produce a slanted smile with his partially paralyzed face. He suspected he looked a sight and wished they had combed his hair before leaving the room.

One of the signs on the entrance read "Nuclear Medicine," and Murph recognized and understood the word "medicine." After a short wait in the X-ray room, yet another doctor, another specialist, introduced himself. The technicians lifted Murph from the wheelchair to the examining table and tilted him into a nearly vertical position. A long tube was pointed at his head and chest. Everyone donned lead aprons—everyone but Murph, that is. Again, Murph felt frightened. As he looked around, he saw Wendy enter the room. Her smile and friendly manner were comforting. To the technicians, Murph was 190 pounds of human mass to be held firmly in position. But to Wendy, he was a person, an individual. At least, that was what Murphy sensed.

Liquid chalk: that's what it tasted like. The barium was a white substance swallowed while a video X-ray was recorded. Wendy and the radiologist watched Murph, Murph's skeleton really, swallow the liquid. Most of it shot down the stomach, but a small amount pooled on the vocal cords. When Murph took another breath, it went directly into his lungs. Murph did better with the barium paste and a cookie soaked in the stuff. But there was no question that Murph breathed the liquid. Wendy noted that, for now, Murph would not be able to eat or drink by mouth and she would recommend that enteral, or tube feeding, should be started.

The tube was coated with K-Y Jelly and slipped through his nose. The nurse kept telling Murphy to "swallow." Actually, she was shouting the word. Once again, Murph wondered if there was something wrong with his hearing. Why would so many people feel the need to shout at him? His nose and throat hurt as the tube went down. Correction. Things don't hurt in a hospital; the patient feels some discomfort. Well, this discomfort hurt! When the end of the tube was finally resting in Murph's stomach and an X-ray was taken, the nurse started feeding Murph through the tube. A white liquid began to flow. This wasn't one of Murph's world class sandwiches, but it was dinner. What was more important, it provided needed liquids and protein. After a while, Murph felt satisfied—not full, but satisfied.

The next day, Murph was moved to the intermediate care unit. In hospital-speak, this is known as a step-down unit. It's not as intense as intensive care, but it's more intense than the acute floor. Murph was beginning to sense there was a definite hierarchy in the hospital world.

Wendy and the other therapists visited him regularly in the intermediate unit. His right arm, leg, and hand were exercised, splinted, ultra-sounded, and massaged. He was taught to stand, sit, and dress differently. Two days later, Murph was moved to the third-floor acute care ward. After learning to chew and swallow more carefully, the tube was pulled from his nose. What a wonderful sensation, almost as good as the taste of the soft food he was given. Soon after that, Murph was transferred to the rehabilitation section of the hospital. He knew something was up when Wendy jokingly said, "The vacation is over."

The fall Murph had taken into the family pictures a few days ago seemed like a distant nightmare. His life had changed permanently. From Murph's perspective, all of the changes were unwanted. In an instant, he was transformed into a dependent, verbally impaired patient in a large, impersonal institution. Although he could see and touch Beth, his mate of 45 years, a wedge had been driven between them. He still felt the love, the fondness for her, but all but the most basic expressions of his feelings were lost. Matt, Andrea, and the grandchildren visited him regularly, but there were painful silences and a lack of friendly chatter. He missed his old life sorely, and it angered him that so much had been taken away. He certainly had not asked for the stroke, but he felt anger at himself for having it. He was frustrated at being unable to change the situation, and angry at the frustration.

The new relationships he had with the hospital staff were even less satisfying. Between exams, punctures, transfers, and drills, communication was a shadow of what it should have been. Murphy felt isolated, lonely, and depressed. Who wouldn't? His depression worsened as the reality of life after stroke set in. The trigger, setting the depressive spiral into motion, was when Murph overheard that the Bounder was for sale. He couldn't understand the details, but it was clear from Beth and Matt's discussion that his Bounder was for sale. Murph slipped deeper and deeper into depression.

Some of Murph's speech and language had returned. This was called spontaneous recovery. Within three weeks of the stroke, Murph's comprehension had returned to the extent that he could understand most of what was spoken to him, as long as people spoke clearly and slowly and avoided complex words. It irritated Murph that some people talked to him like he was retarded. He wasn't, and didn't appreciate being talked to like that. It contributed to his depression. Murph could read short sentences and do some simple arithmetic problems. Each day he was getting better. Most patients who survive a stroke improve, at least somewhat. Words were still forced and slurred when he could find the correct ones, but his speech was now functional, which is hospital-speak meaning he could express his wants and needs. Murph was able to write about as well as he could speak. Wendy told him this was typical for most stroke patients.

Wendy wanted Murph to be put on an antidepressant because he was too depressed, he was devastated beyond a normal grief reaction by the recent events. The injury to the cells of the brain and his inability to adjust to the unwanted events had combined to create a spiral of negativity. The poor guy just couldn't see the light at the end of the tunnel. Wendy would talk to Dr. Curzon about it.

The weekly rehabilitation meetings were highly structured, intense, and always interesting. The physiatrists ran the show and were quite democratic. Each doctor would provide a case history of the patient to be discussed and then call on the respective professionals for their ideas. Wendy sat quietly during the discussion of an 86-year-old woman with a fractured hip and diabetes. Murph was up next, and she wanted to make certain she covered everything in the brief time allotted her.

Dr. Curzon matter-of-factly reviewed Murph's history. "The patient is a 68-year-old male who was transferred to the Rehabilitation Unit three days ago. He is stable and on antibiotics. The thrombosis interrupted blood flow of the middle cerebral artery to the left hemisphere. It was a relatively dense stroke. The patient had hemiparalysis and dysphagia, and was incontinent. He had aspiration pneumonia that is now under control and responding well to the medications."

The physical therapist reported that Murph was doing well. He was still at an "assist level," meaning he was far from being able to walk by himself. Murphy was having trouble transferring from bed to wheelchair and back again. Wendy was delighted to hear that some movement was returning to Murph's right hand. She recalled a lecture of long ago in which the professor reported that speech recovery often correlates with return of function to the right hand.

The occupational therapist reported that Murph was unable to dress himself but was learning self-sufficiency at the expected rate. She noted Murph was not very motivated lately. She explained how Velcro was substituted for zippers and buttons, and that Murph was improving in other ADLs. Activities of daily living were always called ADLs. Wendy was impressed with the tricks of the trade the occupational therapists had. They were quite clever in teaching patients alternative ways of dressing and eating.

The report from the dietician was relatively standard for a stroke patient. Wendy often chuckled to herself when the dietician reported that a particular patient was 10 to 15 pounds over his or her ideal weight. "Who wasn't?" she thought.

The social worker reported that Murph's finances were good. He was in a designated Medicare bed and had supplemental insurance. Out-of-pocket expense would still be considerable, but apparently the family resources could handle it. She noted that Beth was a concerned, caring spouse and was adjusting well to Murph's disabilities. As an aside, she reported Matt tended to be too protective and somewhat anxious about his father. The social worker's final statement was a good introduction to Wendy's presentation. She said Murphy was depressed and becoming more so.

Wendy reviewed Murph's swallowing status. He was on a soft diet and tolerating it well. As long as he took a deep breath before each swallow and paced himself, there were no occurrences of choking or coughing. She was going to advance his diet and stop the Thick-it. Thick-it was a substance put in the patient's liquids to provide more texture. It helped the patient manage thin liquids during swallowing. Thin liquids such as juices and coffee tended to be the most difficult for patients with swallowing problems.

Wendy noted Murph's receptive abilities had improved considerably since her first visit to him in ICU. She reported the results of the Token Test, in which the patient follows commands by pointing to or rearranging differently colored and shaped objects. "Murph can understand the majority of speech. Writing seems to be the modality of communication least improving," she reported.

Wendy noted that programming of the words seemed to be the main difficulty. "Murph," she reported, "has more problems sequencing and planning the utterances than he does in retrieving the words." Both finding the correct name and then being able to plan and program it into existence were problematic. This was the nature of his type of aphasia. She condensed it into the professional jargon everyone at the conference table would understand: "The patient has Broca's aphasia with a predominance of apraxia of speech. He also has mild dysarthria."

Wendy then asked Dr. Curzon if she would consider prescribing an antidepressant for Murphy. She stated that he was extremely depressed, and it was not resolving on its own. She was also concerned at his listlessness and lack of motivation. She thought the antidepressant would help increase his motivation and ability to benefit from therapy. That was the professional rationale provided to Dr. Curzon. Wendy knew the main reason was that Murph was in pain—psychological pain—and it hurt her to see him suffer. In a few days, the antidepressant would kick in and Murph's spirits would elevate. Then, along with the return of more function, he would likely find the strength to adjust to his communication disorders. Too much had gone wrong in this guy's life; too much, too rapidly. Antidepressants provided many patients a leg up on the adjustment process. As a psychologist once told the staff at the rehabilitation meeting, "It's hard to learn to navigate in a storm. The medications calm the seas."

Murph decided Wendy had been right—the time spent in ICU, intermediate, and acute care was a vacation compared to the rehabilitation ward. Everything was structured from morning to night. He was dressed and ready to go by 7:15 a.m. Breakfast was usually taken in his room, although lunch and dinner were held in the communal dining room. By 8:30 a.m., Murph was in the physical therapy gym learning to walk with the assistance of a walker. Things were not going well with the walker. He just couldn't keep his balance. If it weren't for the help of the aide, he would have fallen more than once.

Occupational therapy was helping him become more independent in dressing and feeding himself. He was learning to transfer from his wheelchair to the toilet without falling. Murph had therapy with Wendy twice a day, and he eagerly anticipated the morning and afternoon sessions. The exercises, drills, and games were helping him remember words and ease their production. His facial muscles were becoming stronger; his speech was more precise. The most difficult hurdle to overcome was the tendency of his mouth to have a mind of its own. Some sequences of sounds and certain words were unavailable to him. Try as he would, he just couldn't get the sounds to come out correctly.

"Automatic speech" was a strange phenomenon. Some words and phrases were impossible to speak when he tried to do so. However, when his mind was elsewhere and he wasn't trying to force speech, those words and phrases were spoken easily and articulately. His daughter-in-law's name was a good example. Once in the morning session, Murph was trying to say her name. As he practiced her name, all that came out was "dan rea," "san vea," "dorn a hea." The harder he tried, the more thought he put into it, the further he got from the word. Then, as if in some bizarre magic show, he turned to Wendy and said, "Can't seem to say Andrea today." The automatic utterances were quite frequent and, much to Murph's dismay, readily present on swear words. Murph had never been one to swear much. He was not a crude man. But, boy, the swear words were easy to say since the stroke. They popped out at the worst times, too. He had to work to forget the first words he accidentally said to the minister during his visit. In some ways, automatic speech was a curse.

Wendy had prepared Murph for group. She managed to explain to him that he was going to be provided therapy at the same time as some of the other patients. She wheeled Murphy into the large room and placed the locks on the wheelchair when he was in position at the table.

Across from Murph sat a young man. His head had been shaved and a curious question mark scar was prominent next to his ear. Murph said, "Good morning. My name is Murphy." Actually, Murph said, "Should Morning…name, Murph." He wanted to correct the errors, but Wendy had been clear that the best strategy was to keep going forward in these situations. Too many patients spent too much time revising and correcting, struggling and fighting to make the output perfect. In the world of aphasia, perfection is rarely attainable. She was right. The question mark kid understood what Murph said and replied in a slurred, distorted way.

To Murphy's left was another man. He was about Murph's age. Like Murphy, his arm was also secured to his chest. He nodded when they made eye contact and burst into tears. Murphy knew what was happening; he'd been there, done that. In fact, he was still there, still doing that as he fought to stop his own tears.

Across from the crying man was a woman in her mid-50s. She was a pleasant looking woman who smiled at Murph and said, "Hello, my name is Helen. Welcome to our kroop, stroop." She then opened her mouth widely and carefully said, "group." Murph nodded.

Next to the woman was another man, clearly older than anyone at the table. He just stared out of the window; he didn't acknowledge anyone or anything. He had a blanket wrapped around him, and a tube ran from his nose up to a plastic bag hung on a steel hanger attached to his wheelchair.

Another man walked into the room. At first Murph thought he might be one of the doctors. He waved and nodded to everyone at the table, then turned to Wendy and precisely said, "The chitters have arranged." Now Murph was still having a problem understanding the speech of others, but his was clearly an odd thing for anyone to say. Then the man turned to Murph and followed his observation about the chitters with the statement, "A new chit. Gone a hafta depend on it?" Then the man looked directly into Murph's eyes and awaited a response.

Murph heard a strange sound coming from his throat. It had been a long time since he had last heard it. He was laughing. Laughing out loud. It wasn't Murphy's style to laugh at other people, but this was just too funny. He looked around and all of the patients, except the man in the blanket, were laughing. Wendy seemed to enjoy it the most. When the laughter subsided, Wendy carefully explained to Murph that Mr. Skinner had jargon aphasia. Apparently, the understanding centers of his brain were damaged and he had a degree of denial about the communication disorder. Mr. Skinner believed he was talking normally and people just needed to take the time to understand him. Murphy had a vague recollection of experiencing a similar feeling in the emergency room.

Murph looked forward to group. As time passed, he became friends with Mr. Skinner and the question mark kid. He met the pretty woman's family and tried to build a bridge to the blanket man. But the blanket man was too distant, too alone. Murph hoped he would come around and someday become a participant in group. Murphy learned to accept the group members for who they were, and what they had become. They were all travelers on a difficult road. They all had lost so much. But they were all gaining, too. New friends, new skills.

Beth helped Murph into the old pickup. He noted she had trouble opening the door. He'd have to remember to get some oil for the hinges. With the wheelchair in the back, they drove to their home of 40 years. It was good to be home. He had forgotten how pleasant and predictable a home could be. He managed to get around, mostly in the wheelchair. Matt made the house wheelchair-accessible by building ramps and making two doors wider. Murph still saw Wendy for outpatient therapy three times a week, but at least he was home. Although his speech was far from perfect, he got by. Each day, more words came to him; just like before his fall into the dresser, each new day was an unknown. There would be the good and the bad, the positive and the negative. The stroke had changed many things, but the days continued.

Beth watched Murph playing with the twins in the yard. Murph counted and the twins ran from the fence to a tree. She enjoyed hearing the laughter and screams from the twins. She thought about the Bounder and the trip they would never take. Her thoughts about the motor home and the great cross-country journey were interrupted by the sight of the twins, both of them, hugging their grandpa. Murph was home.

"Murphy's Inner World of Aphasia: Beth's Story," was originally published in *The Family Guide to Surviving Stroke and Communication Disorders* (2nd edition) (Jones and Bartlett Publishers).

On this dark interstate highway, losing one's self in thoughts of roads not taken is so easy. The ever-present engine purr, the whine of steel-belted tires meeting pavement, and the monotony of roadside reflectors sculpt thoughts of long-forgotten days. As Beth drives the Bounder through the dark expanse of southern Arizona, she knows that decisions she made so many years ago mattered. With Murphy sound asleep in the back of the motor home, Beth recalls the lines of a Robert Frost poem she was forced to learn when she was a young school girl:

> *Two roads diverged in a yellow wood,*
> *And sorry I could not travel both*
> *And be one traveler, long I stood*
> *And looked on one as far as I could*
> *To where it bent in the undergrowth;*

When Murph asked for her hand in marriage, he promised life with him would never be boring, a vow that has turned out to be an understatement. Modestly, even to herself, Beth admits there were more handsome, more sophisticated, more polished men vying for her hand, but Murph's cockiness and promise of a lifetime of excitement tipped the marriage equation in his favor. The stroke and aphasia he suffered so many months ago are proving to be the biggest challenge yet, and yes, life is far from boring.

As the motor home purrs through the empty night, Beth realizes the guilt she felt about Murphy's stroke no longer tugs at her conscience. She finally knows, on an important emotional level, that she is not responsible for the plug of something or other that blocked the blood flow to his brain. Strokes happen, and as Dr. Foster said, perhaps nothing could have been done to prevent this life-changing event. Murphy suffered from high blood pressure for several years, but he was exercising, eating better, and religiously taking his medication. Besides, the stroke was not a burst blood vessel that high blood pressure often causes, it was an obstruction.

Sadly for Beth, Murphy, the children and grandchildren, the plug was in the left side of his brain, and it deprived blood to the all-important speech and language centers. As so often happens with strokes affecting speech and language, Murph's right side is also weak, but with the assistance of a quad cane, he can slowly get around. A green freeway sign passing overhead shows the next gas station is 50 miles yonder, and Beth checks the fuel gauge. Relieved that it shows more than half a tank of expensive gasoline remaining, her thoughts briefly return to that terrible morning when Murphy collapsed into the bedroom dresser, knocking the family pictures to the floor. Curiously, she recalls that her first concern was for the broken glass and the potential of cuts, as her mind tried to process the terrible event unfolding before her eyes.

As Beth continues down the road of remembrance, she thinks of her life with Murphy as divided by that disastrous night: before and after aphasia. Certainly, before aphasia, life with Murph was not a cakewalk, and neither was it always an uphill climb. Their early years were full of the stressors all young couples experience as roles, responsibilities, and routines are established. Back then, people married for life, and Beth and Murphy needed time to establish the rules of the lifelong partnership. Beth was thankful Murphy was a communicator; he was never one to hide from her and life in a beer bottle or a televised baseball game. Murphy, at least before the stroke, was not a speechless spectator on life's journey. Although not always pleasant, their communication was open, fair, and giving, and what is most important, they both knew how to listen. The war separated them physically for a time, but they were never far removed from each other's thoughts. Beth never told Murph she kept every war letter in a secret cranny in the very bedroom dresser where the aphasia began. During the worst times in their relationship, she often read them, silently and alone in their sanctuary of their bedroom, as if they were an antidote to the poison threatening their marriage.

They say married couples argue about three things: children, money, and sex. The birth of their children, Matt and Michelle, brought more responsibilities and Murphy and Beth rallied to the occasions. Especially when the children were young, Murphy rarely questioned Beth's rearing habits. When he disagreed, he did so privately and discretely. Beth felt blessed that both children were no more trouble than most, and even during the trying teenage years, home life was usually tolerable.

Looking back, she realizes just how rich their home was in communication. The bantering, arguing, laughing, crying, planning, and even the shouting embodied the energy of their family. And the "love ya" farewells, so naturally uttered as children ran for the school bus, expressed the depth of it all. Communication with the children gradually matured as they grew into young adults. Beth and Murph's directing and protective assertions diminished as the children came of age, and they welcomed Matt and Michelle as adults in the relationship. Beth and Murphy's communication also evolved, with fewer unnecessary words spoken, relying more on mental telepathy to anticipate everything from romance to the passing of a saltshaker. When brainstorming, they appreciated the importance of thoroughly considering an idea without prematurely dismissing it. "Let's run it up the flagpole and see if anyone salutes it" was a common cliché they used when exploring options. Aphasia has now reduced their rich communication to the basics, and it has been many months since Murph has been able to express himself about the important things in life. Beth fancies the harvest moon hanging from the rural Arizona sky and the scent of farmers' crops being readied for market. She pilots the huge recreational machine with confidence and skill while Murphy sleeps quietly, gently rocked by the continuous sway of their temporary home on wheels.

Beth wonders if any couple, other than the suffering super-rich with silver spoons jammed in their mouths, ever has enough money. Beth knows Murph always felt guilty for the constant lack of money they endured despite her frequent assurances. It made matters worse that one of her young suitors has since acquired vast wealth and publicity. Men of Murph's generation took bread-winning seriously, and it didn't matter to Murph's self-esteem that Beth's successful suitor was never a serious factor in the mating equation. The aphasia and the tremendous stroke-related out-of-pocket medical expenses no doubt contributed to Murph's severe clinical depression. Thanks to God, loving family support, therapies, and antidepressants—"happy pills" as the children call them—Murph's spirits have since lifted, at least somewhat. The antidepressants certainly have improved his take on life, but the reality of life after stroke still frequently rears its ugly head. Fortunately, Murph was always an optimist, and even in the depths of his melancholy, Beth could see flickers of his enduring spirit in that silent cavern of despair.

Since Murph's stroke, they have yet to reconnect intimately. They were never a couple to couple incessantly, nor did they engage in public displays of affection, PDAs as their kids say, but they shared a closeness no one else needed to be privy to. It was a physical bridge, but the words they whispered were as much of their love as anything physical. Unlike love in the classic movies of the '40s and '50s, seldom did fireworks light up the sky, nor did symphonies crescendo to their union. Sadly, since the stroke, Murphy has turned away from Beth's soft caresses, apparently shamed by his stroke-ravaged body. What truly saddens Beth about this collapse of the intimacy bridge is that, try as she may, she cannot make him understand that he does not repulse her. Beth also understands that on a deeper level, Murph is just not ready to resume that part of his life. Beth has always been patient about these things, and she will wait until the time is right. After all, when she had her disfiguring breast surgery, Murphy had been there until her self-concept and self-esteem could adapt to the loss. It would be wrong to say that ending their physical intimacy is no big deal, but an exaggeration to deem it an insurmountable obstacle. Beth checks the speedometer to be certain the auto control is keeping the Bounder at the speed limit. For Beth, getting a speeding ticket at her age would be embarrassing and confirm the neighbors' suspicion that the motor home is too much for her handle. "Nonsense," she retorted at the bon voyage party. "I have driven school buses with much more precious cargo and never dented a fender." Beth knows she has never been one mindlessly to step to any drummer's beat as she recalls the second stanza of her favorite poem:

> *Then took the other, as just as fair,*
> *And having perhaps the better claim,*
> *Because it was grassy and wanted wear;*
> *Though as for that the passing there*
> *Had worn them really about the same,*

Murphy's stroke and aphasia have dramatically changed their marital roles, something Beth admits is not necessarily a bad thing. Before aphasia, Murph took care of negotiating mortgages, bargaining with car dealers, trying to get the best value from appliance salespeople, and obtaining credit cards with the lowest interest rates. Beth took care of the usual day-to-day purchases, and gladly deferred to him on the other things, tasks she considered unpleasant. However, six months ago, Beth was thrown into the mix of disagreeable business when their old pickup would not start. In the past, few things were more distressing for Beth than questioning a mechanic's claim that expensive car repairs were necessary. Before the aphasia, Murphy fluently spoke the language of grease monkeys and rarely was he gouged by them. At the auto repair shop, Beth was certain she would not fare well when the mechanic droned on and on about the need for wires, plugs, timing belts, regulators, something called an "alternator," and the thousand dollar price tag it all would carry. He was obviously proud of his special vocabulary, and she was told of the needed parts and labor in a manner typical of a physicist explaining nuclear fusion to a preschooler. Beth surmised what pre-aphasic Murphy would do, and she decided to question the need for each part. Soon it became apparent that a new battery would return the pickup to running status. The mechanic, obviously distressed that a woman would have the audacity to question his vast knowledge of things mechanical, cautioned her that it was just a matter of time until the other repairs would be necessary. He reminded her of the breadth and depth of his mechanical prowess. Beth recalls thinking to herself that everything is just a matter of time, and what matters is how people spend their time. She decided if the pickup became unreliable, she would trade it in on a newer one rather than replace it part-by-expensive-part. The pickup has run just fine since the battery replacement, and Beth smiles when she thinks of driving it from the repair shop, and the mechanic's frown barely hidden beneath grease smudges as he gave her the keys.

Using a small lever on the armrest of the driver seat, Beth adjusts the right rearview mirror and reflects that the worst of the aphasia-times happened immediately after Dr. Foster discharged Murph from the rehabilitation center. Murphy was clearly happy to be released from the confines of the cold, impersonal institution, and to be embraced by the warm familiarity of his home of forty years. After the welcome-home party, when family and neighbors had finally vacated the premises, Beth and Murph sat quietly in the living room. There was an awkwardness to the moment much like strangers feel on an elevator while making small talk. Murph occasionally gave her that slanted smile she had grown accustomed to in the hospital, and several times he telegraphed shortened utterances Beth could not clearly decipher. He apparently wanted to express something very profound. They danced the dance of aphasia, and in the end, communication failed them. It was an extremely frustrating moment, and for the first time in their relationship, Beth was strangely uncomfortable around him. She was not uncomfortable with Murph per se; she was ill at ease with her thoughts about the future and dealing with his disabilities. She sensed that Murph was shamed by his childlike speech. She sensed he shuddered at the thought of another bout of incontinence and the necessity of adult diapers. She sensed he felt diminished as a man and dreaded being a lifelong burden. She sensed he feared for the future and would welcome an end to it all. And what disturbed Beth most about this awkwardness was that she sensed Murph might be right. Fortunately, Beth recalls as she passes a lumbering cross-country tractor-trailer truck with an insufficient hill-climbing engine, her appraisal of the situation was unduly pessimistic. She whispers the third stanza of Robert Frost's immortal refrain:

> *And both that morning equally lay*
> *In leaves no step had trodden black.*
> *Oh, I kept the first for another day!*
> *Yet knowing how way leads on to way,*
> *I doubted if I should ever come back.*

The doctors call it spontaneous recovery, and it occurs in most stroke patients. It is the natural tendency of the body to heal itself, and when combined with therapies, many patients improve significantly in their physical and communication abilities. Fortunately, Murphy was one of the lucky ones, and his walking and talking improved over time. His expensive wheelchair is now parked in the guest bedroom, at least for now. The Americans with Disabilities Act is most helpful for Murphy, and millions like him. Nowadays, there are plenty of handicapped parking spaces, ramps, and specially constructed elevators and bathrooms. Thanks to that landmark legislation, disabled people are far less handicapped and can continue to participate fully in life despite their limitations. Beth and Murphy have been pleasantly surprised to find that other travelers, for the most part, are also kind and patient with the disabled. Food servers, ticket takers, ushers, and other service people also take the time and have the necessary patience when dealing with Murphy's new life challenges.

Beth has been careful to walk a fine line between expecting too much and too little of her post-stroke husband. Expecting too much sows the seeds of frustration and failure, and what is even worse, ultimately blows to his frail self-esteem. Beth knows Murph is talking as well as he can and that hurrying him, or demanding communication perfection, disrupts the process even more. On the other hand, expecting too little of Murphy condemns him to a lifetime of victimization and promises unrealized. Each day, Beth walks that tenuous fine line.

As Beth returns the Bounder to the right lane, she ponders the decisions she and Murphy have made since aphasia entered their lives. They could have become victims to the stroke and aphasia, given up, and succumbed to the inevitable. Beth could have studied brochures of nursing homes and assisted living centers, and sought relief from her uncommunicative burden. For pessimists, that would certainly be the sanest course of action for a woman her age. Murph could have refused therapies and resigned himself to the multitude of losses the aphasia hath wrought. After all, everyone knows there comes a time to accept disabilities rather than mindlessly trying to overcome them. The children and grandchildren could have turned back from their aphasic patriarch and the flimsy bridge of communication connecting them, and bid their father and grandfather farewell. They could have heeded the advice of friends and family and gone through with the sale of the Bounder. This marvelous traveling machine could be in the hands of a different couple traveling life's roads. Perhaps the philosophical mechanic was right; it really is just a matter of time, and the "sooner the better." Then, just perhaps, the mechanic was wrong on both counts.

Beth knows she and Murph were never easy victims; they have always confronted life's challenges with determination and persistence. Beth knows that accepting the losses aphasia brought to their lives is different from being resigned to them. Stroke and aphasia are major life events, but at least for Beth and Murphy, they are not sufficient to detour them from enjoying the many roads yet to be traveled in the sunset of their lives. Beth again checks the fuel gauge and realizes that there still is plenty of gasoline to get them to parts unknown. The freeway sign shows a historical detour to a town called "Tombstone" and a daily reenactment of a gunfight at an OK Corral. The signal light beeps, beeps, beeps as the Bounder exits the well-worn freeway and Beth recites aloud the final stanza of Robert Frost's famous ode to roads not taken:

> *I shall be telling this with a sigh*
> *Somewhere ages and ages hence:*
> *Two roads diverged in a wood, and I-*
> *I took the one less traveled by,*
> *And that has made all the difference.*

Alternately Abled

"Alternately Abled" was originally published in *The Psychology of Neurogenic Communication Disorders: A Primer for Health Care Professionals* (Pearson Allyn & Bacon Publishers).

Chapter One

Sometimes, you misjudge people. It is so easy to jump to conclusions, so comfortable to rely on tried and true stereotypes no matter how untested they are. Prejudices are natural, you know. We "prejudge." When sitting on a chair, you know it will hold your weight because in the past, thousands of chairs have saved your butt from crashing to the floor. You expect the sun to rise in the morning because it has peeked over the horizon every day since there were eyes to witness the explosion of light and color. You prejudge your car's stopping power on icy roads, the wince and watery eyes from too many drops of Tabasco sauce, and the certainty that your dog will keep running even when you demand its halt. You are unconsciously certain that electrons will reach the bulb when you grope for the light switch early in the morning; they will because they have. We must prejudge; our sanity relies on it. The world would be a frighteningly chaotic blur if the past did not foretell the future.

It is our prejudices about people that muck up the works. Two rude blond waitresses and you expect the third to be surly. A criminal markup of parts and labor by one mechanic and you expect the same from all grease monkeys. Being mugged by a young man with baggy pants and tattoos of snakes alerts your nighttime senses to all males, loose-fitting pants and reptilian body art. Prejudices about people are the same type of generalization, the same process of predicting the future, but sometimes they are fraught with error.

I did everything I could to keep the Cessna in the air, to keep it flying. From the time I heard the sickening clunk and grinding of pistons and bearings gone awry, I went by the book. In the world of aviation, every eventuality has been anticipated and there are rules for dealing with them. That's what "flying by the book" means. I tried to restart the engine. Three times I tried to get the propeller to turn, but it seemed frozen— super-glued in place. The only sound was the whoosh of the air as the dead plane began to drop from the sky. The passengers were quiet and frozen like the plane's engine. I looked for a flat, smooth place to land, but Alaska is a rugged place. The river, winding through the deep canyon, seemed the least of the landing evils. A water landing would be bad, but not nearly as disastrous as shooting through pine trees.

Yes, I was frightened, but there was little time and too much to do to be consumed by fear. I knew I would do my best and with luck, save my life and the lives of my passengers. As the trees and river rapidly approached, I shut off the fuel. In the microphone of my Sony headset, I announced our impending doom to anyone and everyone. On the emergency band, I declared every pilot's worst fear: "Cessna three four four five niner, May Day, May Day. Lost power, crash landing into Dolores River. Cessna three four four five niner, May Day, May Day."

I heard some whimpering and quiet sobbing from the passengers, but much to their merit, there was no panic, no shouting, and no screaming. I told them to tighten their seat belts and shoulder harnesses, to cover their faces with their hands, and to get out of the plane as soon as possible when we were on the ground. I also said we were going to make it; we were going to walk away from this landing. Little did they know that it was said more for my benefit than theirs.

We were a long way from anyone. Alaska can be desolate. I knew even if we survived the landing, getting home would be an equally challenging feat.

I said into the headset, "Cessna three four four five niner, May Day, May Day. Lost power, crash landing into Dolores River." I then "squawked" my identification by pressing 34459 on my instrument panel, hoping it would light up our position, speed, direction, and other valuable information on the Fairbanks tower's radar screen. "Cessna three four four five niner, May Day, May Day. I'm about 130 miles north, northeast of Tuktoyuktuk. Cessna three four four five niner, May Day, May Day."

Gravity continued to pull us down until I could clearly see the pine cones hanging from the tops of trees. I fought the reflex to pull back on the yoke; to try to make the airplane climb from the approaching danger. I kept the nose down and the speed up. I aimed for the smoothest part of the choppy river and shouted "Hang on, brace yourselves" to the passengers. I turned the main power switch to "off." Then, a calm fell over me. It is the kind of feeling you get when you realize that you've done your best and everything is now in the hands of God and fate. There are no more decisions, no more options. Life and death will play out, and I was just an observer to the unfolding events. About ten feet above the water, I pulled up the nose of the plane and tried for a controlled stall, to stop in midair, and gently drop to safety.

Unbelievably cold. The water was freezing and it numbed my senses. I was disoriented and couldn't tell up from down. I swallowed and choked on cold, blood-soaked Alaskan water. My lungs ached and demanded oxygen. Something twisted and red pinned my right leg, and I couldn't free it. I was flailing, struggling to free myself, but I really wasn't panicked. I was resigned to my watery fate and the struggle was just an act—something my body needed to do. All I could hear was the muffled roar of the river. Just as I started to lose consciousness, I felt two strong hands tug, jerk and pull my pinned leg. There was a little movement, then more, and finally I broke free from the death grip. Those same strong hands grabbed the lapels of my flight jacket and pulled me through the small crumpled door of the Cessna. Through the cold, clear Alaska water, I could see a round face wince as he struggled to push me to the surface. My rescuer was the heavy set one. My lifesaver was one of the passengers. As I broke through the surface of the river, and sucked in the wonderful fresh Alaskan air, I realized I had been saved by one of the retarded passengers. My savior was one whom I had dismissed, felt superior to, and made jokes about. It was the good-natured one. I owed my life to him. He had risked his, dove beneath the surface, forced himself through the small opening, and freed my leg. And he did it with four broken ribs and a nasty slash on his shoulder and back. Sometimes, you misjudge people.

Chapter Two

I love this campus and its hundreds of grassy, green acres dotted by huge oak and maple trees, flowering bushes, and small, manicured gardens. Thousands of students swarm this academic sanctuary, busily rushing from one class to another, to and from the library complex and home to dingy dorms and apartments. Sometimes I sit on one of the iron benches outside the International Center and just take in the sights, sounds, smells and energy that is this large Midwestern university. I study the young and not-so-young men and women confidently pursuing their studies with the hope that their future will be better because of it. It's called "delayed gratification." It is the act of putting off house, Corvette, garden, profession, and family until the four, six, or eight years of study are complete. It's the belief that all will work out for the best and those years of timed tests, teaching, and tutoring will pay off. It is the belief that the pay will be not just in money, but also in quality of life. Higher education is a promise our society makes to the intelligent. And usually the promise is fulfilled. Education is good.

There are so many different types of people soaking up the rich education this campus has to offer. Bearded young men with very intense faces, jocks with fancy cars and bruised bodies, granolas and tree huggers, sorority sisters, stoners, young republicans, cowboys, and debaters. There are thespians, always on stage and making grand entrances, medical students haughtily burdened by huge books on pathology and pediatrics, future lawyers planning and scheming to get the biggest slice of the American pie, aspiring accountants, psychologists, and managers. I know I should be sent to a nauseating sexual harassment workshop, but I enjoy watching the women. I watch them walk, sit, smile, and be. As I ride this diesel-coughing bus to my office, I study them. I particularly like women who wear glasses. I wonder about the hot, sensual ways hidden behind their librarian facade. She just smiled at me, eyes sparkling, legs crossed, breasts present. It sends my heart into arrhythmia, and I can feel the blood rush to my face.

Of course, my thoughts of her are pure fantasy with nary the slightest chance of becoming reality. You see, I'm a gimp. Cerebral palsy has given me the walk and talk of a pitiful person. I have these crutches to help me get from here to there, but I'm clumsy, awkward and slow. I have spastic muscles constantly fighting and pulling against each other. My voice is raspy and my speech is slow. It seems I'm constantly repeating myself to the "what" "pardon," and "huh" of my listeners. It gets frustrating and sometimes downright infuriating. I know I have a good mind. I am a professor, after all, with diplomas and an academic gown to prove it. I was told by my high school sweetheart that I also have a good personality. If the sensual librarians would get to know me, they would see I am passionate about my passions, quick-witted and thoughtful. I've got a great imagination probably because I need one. So many things are out of reach for me physically, but I can soar in my mind. In my mind, the sweet, sensual librarian is lying exhausted on the sweat soaked bed, flush-faced, begging me to return as I dress, look for my car keys and hurry off to my 10:00 a.m. course. Thank God for an imagination and women who wear glasses.

I must keep my fantasy flights about librarians secret. If I were normal physically, I suppose some women would find them a turn-on. If I were normal physically, most men would chuckle, realizing that this is how real men think. It's a guy thing, and the politically correct might just as well try to stop the wind from blowing as to bring an end to these fantasy romps. But, as a gimp with slow and awkward speech, I'd better keep them to myself. For normal men, they are as natural as breathing, but for me they're a perversion. Sex and the disabled are taboo. It's something about the gene pool and propagating the best and fittest. I sure as hell had better keep my flights of fantasy a secret from my girlfriend, Janet. I'd be looking for more than my car keys if I shared my librarian secrets with her.

The closest bus stop to my office is about a thousand yards. A thousand yards doesn't seem like much to someone with strong legs and a normal body, but for me, it's a challenge, especially when there are snow and ice to deal with. We had a late-spring snow about a week ago, and there are still ice spots dotting the sidewalk. After the bus pulled away and the cloud of diesel lifted, I began my shuffle. First the metal cane attached to my right-hand finds a secure spot then I shift my weight to it and drag and slide forward. Next, my left hand performs the same act of locomotion and off I go, each step showing the strain on my face. Plop-slide, plop-slide, plop-slide. Hundreds of students and a fat, bearded colleague float by me, not making eye-contact and hurrying to their destinations.

A thousand yards is about three football fields, and like a star halfback, I go from goal to goal dodging people and things while the crowd cheers. When I get to the door of the Arts and Science Annex, I must push the large, blue handicapped button for it to open. Today, a middle-aged woman, tall and slender, smiles at me, and pulls it open. She has large, dark eyes and darker skin, and very short hair, showing off her long, sensual neck. I like long, sensual necks. As I plop and slide through the opened door, I detect a wisp of strawberry or sage. I slur a "thank you," and muster a smile at her kindness. Several students stand to the side allowing me enough room to park a semi. As I continue forward on the gray and white checkered tile, I hear her whisper a loving, adoring song: "Be careful Ben. I'll wait forever if necessary." Then, as I bravely begin the rescue of the children, assault rifle strapped to my strong back and determination on my rugged, handsome face, I hear her shout: "I love you." Dramatic marching music plays in my ear as I risk life and limb for the children held by evil terrorists.

"We need to talk." In an abrupt flash, I am jolted back to reality by the sound of Janet's voice. I see her sitting on a chair next to my office door.

Janet and I have been together for seven years. The more time I spend with her the more I love her. She's intelligent, beautiful, and compassionate. She has long, jet-black hair and her skin is fair and smooth. She has the kind of smile that brightens up the darkest room, and you can get lost in her eyes. I've never had the courage to ask her why she chose to be with me, what with all the normal, handsome men in the world preening and strutting for her attention. I've seen their eyes follow her as she walked down a hall or out of a room. Physically, she's like a magnet, and her personality is even more seductive. The closest I have come to understanding her willingness to be with me was when I asked her why she chose to work with the disabled. After all, she could be a smartly dressed executive, lunching and planning corporate policy to smartly dressed subordinates who hang on her every word. In the corporate world, she could have had all of the trappings of power, money, and success. But the path she took is cluttered with concrete thinking, drooling, seizures, acting out, slurred speech, and frustration. Her answer to my question was typically to the point: "It's just what I do."

I keep my office tidy. It's not that I am a tidy person, it is just that ambient junk can cause a gimp like me to fall to the hard floor. So, I'm a tidy person by necessity, not by an ordered mind. Janet sat in the small couch donated to the Center where she works. I bought it for $20.00 and it was delivered by Elroy and Nick, two of the strongest residents at the Center. Both have Down syndrome and are in their twenties. I like them both, but I like Elroy the most. Elroy is a very thoughtful person, in his own way. I know he has the hots for Janet and he does little to hide it. When he is around her he blushes, fumbles, and befuddles. He adores her, as do I. I've resolved that if he gets any bolder about her,

I might have to kick his befuddled butt. That would be a sight, he and I fighting for the hand of the damsel.

"They funded it. The grant came through," Janet announced with that soft, sensual voice that turns me to jelly. About a year ago, she applied for a grant from a private foundation for a field trip for some of the residents of the Center. According to excited Janet, Horizons (a privately-held philanthropic organization) funded, in total, the trip to Alaska. Five members of the Center along with Janet and I would jet to Anchorage and then to Fairbanks. Then, a bush pilot would fly us to a fishing and hunting cabin where we would experience the great outdoors to develop character and independence. When she was writing the grant, I thought the whole idea was crazy. What organization in its right mind would donate, with no strings attached, thousands of dollars for a wilderness trip for a bunch of defectives? Apparently Horizons would, and they didn't bat an eye. Thanks to Horizons, we would have this great Alaskan adventure.

The Center for Human Development is located west of the university, on State Street. The Center is made of red brick with window and door frames painted white. Actually, there are three buildings and a grassy green area the residents call the "park." The administrative building is the smallest of the three structures but has the finest office equipment, carpet, and furniture. The dormitory building consists of sixteen apartments, each specially designed for mentally and physically impaired dwellers. There is also a dining room in the basement. The industrial shop and retail store are where business is conducted. People can purchase donated furniture, clothing, lamps, toys, office equipment, small and large appliances, books, and a host of other discarded, tax-deductible items in the store. All of the goods are sorted, cleaned, repaired, and made presentable by the mentally and physically defective residents and the supervisors of the facility. Those with the lowest IQs sort and hang clothing. The ones with higher-functioning but still defective minds do various other tasks to make the goods saleable. The Center also contracts with apartments and businesses to clean and manicure their grounds. Some of the residents have regular eight-to-five jobs and are hustled off every morning to coffee shops, restaurants, and industrial parks in a white stretch van with the Center's name proudly painted on the doors. Janet is Director of Vocational Services and is loved by everyone at the Center, especially Elroy.

Chapter Three

Lunch break at the Center is like free time at any blue-collar place of employment. Some of the women sit at a table, talk and eat from brown bags. Other workers lie on soft bundles of clothing, sleeping or just resting their eyes. A young couple eats together in a secluded corner of the lounge making small talk, laughing and planning their future. A radio blasts tunes in the warehouse while several young men play touch football. Elroy crouches behind a center grunting "Hut one, hut two, hut three" and finally takes the ball from a man who has no idea what a "hut" or a "three" is. Elroy drops back, plants his feet firmly and throws a short pass to a 30-year-old man with a mental age of eight. He manages to catch the ball but is immediately tagged by a buck-toothed linebacker with a serious drooling problem. Don't most linebackers have drooling problems? Two college women, donning the first skimpy shorts of spring, walk past the large warehouse doors between the two parked trucks and "time" is called. The football players watch them meander down the sidewalk and a few men make the type of comments heard at most construction sites from burly, hardhats who think a catcall is the same as foreplay. Has any woman ever stopped, walked back to the hardhats and found them irresistible? Yes, lunch break at the Center is like free time at any blue-collar place of employment.

Elroy watches Ben and Janet enter the administrative offices. Seeing Janet brightens his day. Immediately, he calls an end to the ball game and walks toward the administration building. The players, quizzical looks on their faces, mill around, wonder what happens next. Elroy's mind quickly conjures a reason to talk to her. Of course his motives are transparent to all with IQs above seventy. All Elroy is aware of is the pressing need to hear her voice, see her smile and maybe, just maybe, to be touched by her soft, warm, feminine hands. She often grasps his arm or strokes his shoulder when discussing his phony, made-up topics. Actually, Elroy isn't much more awkward than an average ten-year-old male with a crush on an older woman. After all, Elroy is really just a ten-year-old in a body that has aged twenty-six years.

"Do we need to lock up?" Elroy asks as he stands too close to her. Janet immediately stops walking and smiles, "Of course, but not now, Elroy." Had Elroy a tail, it would have wagged. He looks at Ben and snortingly replies: "Not now." In Elroy's world, he has taken Janet away from his rival and through sheer cunning won the competition for her heart. She is now with him, torn away from Ben. Her warmth is all his and he lords it over Ben. His grin and eye-contact clearly say: "Take that, Professor." In the world of sub average IQs, Janet has chosen him and the relationship will last forever. Score one for the home team.

In the conference room, Janet makes the announcement to the five lucky residents. Four of them, along with Ben, sit on steel folding chairs. Elroy sits next to Janet on the edge of a conference table, basking in her warmth, clearly the dominant male with his prize. Next to Ben is Anastasia. Her life at the Center began with her mother's drinking problem. Anastasia's case history said her mother died of alcoholism in her mid-forties. Actually, the cause of death was listed as an automobile accident late one Saturday night.

But her death was really caused by wine coolers and scotch chasers. She was a binge drunk, and during one of her binges, Anastasia was born. For eight months before her birth, Anastasia developed in an alcohol-saturated womb. It left her frail, frightened, and mentally deficient. Even now, as she approaches nineteen, Anastasia's life is a hangover. When she reaches out, which is not often, Anastasia speaks slowly and rarely understands complicated instructions. She is also prone to temper tantrums. She works at the most menial jobs, the ones that require the least of her deficient problem-solving abilities. Anastasia's job at the Center is to sort hangers. She sees to it that wire, blue, yellow, and white hangers are placed with their own kind.

Autism wreaked havoc on Rusty's young parents eighteen years ago; Rusty appeared normal at first. He nursed, crawled, and cried like most babies. His mother, an only child herself, thought all was well until her nagging suspicions were confirmed by specialists. As Rusty grew to toddle, he became more distant and aloof. Often, he treated his loving parents as objects in the same detached manner as he did his mechanical toys. But it was the echolalia that frightened them. Most normal children go through a stage of speech development where they repeat what has been spoken. But Rusty did it all of the time and never outgrew it. He also liked to see the light flicker when he strobed his fingers close to his eyes. Echoed speech, hand stimulation, and a tendency to rock back and forth had led to Rusty's life at the Center. It was all too much for the loving parents and when their marriage collapsed, Rusty had nowhere to go. But he was soon to go to Alaska and experience the great outdoors, and perhaps, find an escape from his shell.

The other two adventurers are becoming an item at the Center. Trevor and Nicole, both seventeen, are feeling the teenage chemistry. They both have a fondness for fruit punch and it was at the soft drink machine where they began. Trevor is borderline in his intelligence and has the endearing manner of Forrest Gump. Nicole had fallen head-over-heels in love with him. Trevor has begun to return her love, but it is taking time. It simply takes more time for Trevor to process life. He isn't put off by her deformed back and legs. In fact, he finds her physically irresistible, especially her young breasts. They mesmerize him. Two weeks ago, she had let him touch them. After "lights out," she had quietly knocked at his apartment door and they had slipped to the basement, finding the large linen closet unlocked and inviting. Nothing was said as she removed her blouse and unfastened her bra. She took his hands, and for the first time, Trevor touched them. Electricity shot through their bodies as they kissed and caressed. Body heat rose and there was an uncontrollable, primal need to be closer, to be one. But a car's alarm system frightened the young lovers and abruptly ended the passion. In the staff parking lot, the honk, honk, honk brought an early end to their exploration. They returned to their respective floors without being caught, determined that there would be a next time—and soon. That night, they both lay on their beds, reliving the passion, their hearts resonating the intensity of young love.

Chapter Four

Autumn is my favorite season, but spring ranks second. In spring, trees return to life, flowers bloom, grass turns green, and the days get longer. I need longer days. I need sunshine. I get moody and depressed during the winter when the days are short and the sky overcast. In the dark, dreary months of winter, my problems seem bigger, my frustrations greater, and my cerebral palsy more handicapping. I just don't feel good. I eagerly anticipate Spring Break. For many of the students on this campus, Spring Break is a long car ride to Florida, Mexico, or Arizona. Their time is full of beer, and one-night stands. But, for me, Spring Break signals the end of wintry dark and the brightness of renewal. I've done Spring Break Ritual once, but I seemed to be an observer rather than a participant. My buddies were good about helping me get around, finding plenty of room for my crutches, and listening politely while I droned on. But they won the girls, drank the beer and puked the poison from their bodies over the balcony of the motel room. They spent the night in the drunk tank and barely remembered the brawl. Oh, I wanted to win the girls, but with so many tanned, normal male bodies it just wasn't in the cards. What woman would want to boast of a romp with a gimp? How seductive can you be with spastic speech? I drank a few beers but I'm tipsy enough without them. Besides, I have to be careful with alcohol because the more I drink, the less disabled I am. After a six pack or so I'm superman, but much more handsome and with a wonderful ability to sing. In fact, I sang, "Buh, Buh, Bad to the Bone," while my buddies brawled. Well, someone had to.

I teach literature. It is my calling in life. When I lecture to large classrooms of students, sometimes I lose myself in Hemingway, Steinbeck, Ruston, Hillerman, and MacDonald. I may be physically imperfect, slow of speech, and clumsy of body, but when my mind is saturated with literature, I become one with its glory and perfection. Sometimes students sense my rapture and join me in the depth of thought that is literature. I love it. I even like reading their papers. Oh, I know most have only read the Cliffs Notes, but every now and then a sophomore from a farming community or a tenement in the projects will connect with a great writer's mind and story. She will sense the writer's marvelous ability to turn a phrase, and in turn, capture something profound about the human condition. Then she too will turn a phrase, sometimes as eloquent as the writer's, and teleport those insights to me in the form of a twelve-page paper, double-spaced and carefully spell-checked. Unfortunately, with scores of papers to grade, I can only note my pleasure at her growth with a brief statement made with red ink, apply an "A" to her new and hard-fought insights, and move onto the next paper in the foot-high stack.

Spring term rolled along, and as the great Alaskan adventure approached, both Janet and I began to plan for the trip. It's true, the Devil, not God, is in the details. Tickets for Alaska were purchased and the airline told of the special needs of its passengers. Permission forms were completed by parents and guardians, and boots and raincoats purchased. Hours were spent on the telephone to Anchorage, Fairbanks, and bush pilots. The weather channel was watched intently to see what was typical for that part of the huge state of Alaska. Several times Janet and I both confessed that we may have bitten off more than could be chewed. The Alaskan adventure would bring out the best and worst of all of us. It would test our mettle.

Chapter Five

Watching them laugh, share bites of sandwiches and chocolate bars, and touch each other's arms and thighs, Janet knew the time had come. Nicole and Trevor had moved to the next level, and things needed to be done. Birth control was going to be necessary, and perhaps it was already too late. Janet was matter-of-fact about these things. It wasn't a question of morality, it was one of reality. Janet was not a fuddy-duddy. The reality was that without birth control, soon Nicole and Trevor would bring another life into this world. Not that there was anything wrong with that; they had every right, even a biological obligation, to begin their lives together and to have children. It was simply a matter of timing and choice. They were both too young, and for them, because of their disabilities, special plans needed to be made before they jumped into the rest of their lives and the responsibilities of a new one. Things needed to be thought out and not left to chance and the back seat of a car. Janet and Melissa, another counselor at the Center, would take the initiative, make the appointments, and do the counseling. All of this had to be done quietly, almost secretively. People don't like the idea of sex and the disabled. It makes them uncomfortable. It makes some people ugly.

Janet had been with the Center for twelve years. It was her first professional job after graduating from the University with a Master's in Rehabilitation Counseling. Her primary job was to find employment for residents of the Center. She was very lucky. She was also very persuasive in showing their abilities rather than their disabilities. Some of them worked in the auto-parts plant sorting nuts, bolts, and screws and placing them in small, plastic packages. Some bussed tables, mopped floors, and placed dirty dishes in washing machines. One of the residents, a middle-aged man with many disabilities including deafness, worked next to a noisy industrial mixer while it ground and combined rocks and chemicals. Prolonged noise exposure was not a problem for him, and he didn't need to wear sweaty ear plugs and muffs. Sometimes it surprised Janet just how accommodating businesses were, and it wasn't because of welfare, or government projects like Affirmative Action or the Americans with Disabilities Act. It was business, the bottom line, and the fact that the disabled were the best fit for many jobs. Society had come a long way from the time when her people stood on corners, hats in hand, begging for food and money. Some say the label "handicapped" came from those days.

Janet loved the residents of the Center. All of them. Well, most of them. There were two who got on her nerves; a boy and woman she found difficult to like, let alone love. She had to admit, she felt no guilt about her negative feelings for them. We don't live in a perfect world and there was nothing that required her to love them all. She took people one at a time. Their race, gender, religion, and preferences were not as important as their individuality. Janet processed people individually. The woman was in her forties and was unpleasantly bossy and arrogant. She was also dismissive toward Janet. She had the personality traits Janet found herself wanting to avoid. She found herself avoiding the boy, too. Ron frightened her. He was big, reckless, and out of control, and the medications didn't seem to help. Several times he had struck other residents, causing bloody noses and bruised eyes. Each time there was no remorse or promise never again to let frustration turn to violence. To Janet, he was a disaster waiting to happen. He frightened her. The residents had begun to call him "Bad Ron."

Janet went back to her office to make the call to Planned Parenthood. She was one of the few staff members with walls. The others lived and worked in cubicles. She prided herself on the tasteful way she decorated those walls. The decor included ferns and flowers, not too small or large, a small maple table rather than a cold, metal desk, and a wooden filing cabinet. She had only one picture, tastefully framed and strategically placed on her table-desk. It was of her, Ben, and their pug, Rosie. It was an action snapshot of their lives rather than a posed, artificial one. It showed them boarding Ben's specially-equipped van and was taken by their neighbor, a retired professor with a photography hobby. Pugs, perhaps the ugliest animals in the kingdom, take great pictures. They are natural showoffs. Ben takes a good one, too. And except for needing to lose ten or fifteen pounds, so did she. For the past five years, Janet knew she was going to lose those excess hip pounds, and soon. She even put off buying new outfits, knowing they would be too baggy, what with her new diet and all.

Janet had met Ben in college and it wasn't love at first sight. She had learned from the past that love at first sight usually required a second look. The man before Ben had been handsome and cocky. It was the cockiness she had found attractive. He was self-assured, convinced of his ability to succeed at anything and everything. They dated for three years, off and on. About two years into the relationship, Janet realized he was still looking beyond her for something or someone. She also knew she was still shopping, and he hadn't proven himself worthy. Janet prided herself on her high standards for a mate and a father of her yet-to-be-conceived children. She wouldn't settle for just handsome and cocky; there had to be substance. And then she met Ben.

Janet often thought of Ben during her jogs. Early morning jogs had become yet another arsenal in the battle of the bulge around her hips. Actually, Janet could have been a starved Ethiopian poster child and she still would have jogged early in the mornings. She loved the early-morning quiet, crisp air, and the sun rising, bringing a new day of possibilities. She didn't jog far, just two miles around the southern end of the campus and into the small unincorporated township. The campus and city planners created a wonderful maze of jogging trails with rustic wooden bridges, a tunnel, arrows, bright yellow halogen lights, and yield signs. The path she usually pounded coursed through the campus and along Oak River, where ducks, muskrats, and turtles the size of boulders slipped beneath the muddy Midwestern water. There were the usual early-morning joggers pacing themselves to rapid, deep breathing. Like ships in the night, they would cross paths or overtake each other, and nod or simply utter, "morning." By D-day, July 5th, the day they would leave for Anchorage, Janet hoped to have doubled her distance, endurance, and strength.

As Janet rounded the bend and crossed the first of three bridges, she pondered Ben and how to break the news. Janet wanted a child. She wanted the intimacy of an infant, the smell of talcum powder, dirty diapers, breast feeding, tricycles, and the energy of a toddler. She wanted PTA meetings, Christmas concerts, 8th-grade sock hops, prom dresses, and wedding plans. She wanted to be a mother. Nature was nudging, and the time was right. If the past seven years had proven anything, it was that she and Ben could do the family thing. Ben would be a great father, loving yet firm, and he would succeed at hunting and gathering. The Center even had a family-leave policy that would allow Janet an uninterrupted year to nest. Together, they would create a wonderful home for a lucky boy or girl.

In the past, Ben had been reluctant to talk of children. He managed to change the subject whenever it was broached. They talked of everything and anything, and Ben was characteristically open, except about babies and children. A few months ago, Janet realized Ben was afraid. Janet knew Ben and admired his tenacity. Fear was not a big part of his life, but she sensed it when the conversation turned to children. Why he was fearful was beyond her comprehension.

Ben was a good man. Oh, Janet realized that was not saying much. Men are men, and Ben, like most of them, didn't have a clue. The good ones are intelligent, open, caring, committed, and loving. The good ones laugh easily. But the good ones think too much like the not-so-good ones. They think it's all about strength, size, power, appearance, and bravado. The good women, and Janet knew she was one, were more thoughtful about life, love, and relationships. Her love for Ben had begun in a class they shared in graduate school and gradually blossomed. Each day, their relationship strengthened. He had the little things that are so important. He had the important day-to-day things that made their relationship. Ben was a good man, but he didn't have a clue. Even when they fought, he fought fair, and hurtful remarks were kept to a minimum. When the fighting became too much, he simply got in his van and drove to nowhere in particular. Only once had a fight threatened their relationship. Afterward, the emotionally battered combatants had simply returned home and resolved to never let it go too far again. It frightened them.

Janet's pace picked up as she thought more intently about the important things in life. She entered the brightly lit tunnel, which was dug beneath a bicycle path, and heard her expensive running shoes slap the track and echo from the red brick walls. Maybe, she thought, Ben wasn't ready. Maybe it was just that he needed time to get comfortable with the idea. For Janet, time was running out. Unlike men, women hear the distant biological clock ticking away uterine opportunities. Janet could hear the clock, and she knew time was running out. Life is timed, like all of the tests she took in college. For Janet, the time had come.

Chapter Six

I suppose it is because professors make it look easy. Lecturing looks easy, but it is not. It's demanding, hard work. It can go bad in the blink of an eye. Mine usually go well, but sometimes the clock on the wall crawls on, students appear as decaying zombies, PowerPoint or overheads die, and a student with a cold and a honking cough can require more repetitions than usual. Because of my speech disorder, I usually use a microphone, but sometimes it dies, too, and there is always the problem with high-pitched feedback. Sometimes, it's all about motivation. I wake up and would just as soon not talk to anyone, let alone a classroom of seventy-five curious minds. Lecturing can also be exhilarating, especially when exploring an author famous for his or her insight and wit. It can be the best of times and it can be the worst of them. Lecturing can be a rush.

Janet and I rarely fight or even argue. We did more of it when our relationship was young. I suppose it is because we were staking territory and learning boundaries. I don't know if it is by design or chance, but Janet usually prompts an argument about an hour before my lectures. She announces "Round One" of these emotionally draining events by saying, "We need to talk." This is woman speak for, "You're in trouble now." True to form, about an hour before my 2:20 p.m. lecture, over ham and cheese sandwiches, she, out of the blue, simply announced that she didn't want to refill her birth control prescription, and that "We need to talk." Of course, she caught me in mid swallow, and when you have spastic speech muscles, swallowing is also difficult. So, after five attempts to push the mouthful down my dry throat, I was finally able to respond, and it was a pretty pathetic response: "Huh?" What's a guy to say about that type of an announcement? And besides, Janet already knew how this discussion would turn out. She had already planned and predicted the outcome. All she was doing was bringing me up to speed, informing me of this major change in my tenuous life. See, I'm not as dumb as I look.

Right now, I need a pregnant mate like I need another neuromuscular disorder. Hell, let's have a baby and give me multiple sclerosis, too. I'm already off the scale on the stress index. We're not just talking about a baby here. Actually, I'd like a little curtain climber and rug rat brightening up my life. But I know Janet. We're also going to get married. Who'd want to have a child without the benefit of marriage? We're also going to have to get a larger apartment or even our own house. You couldn't raise a child in this one-bedroom dump. Of course, "Mother," my soon-to-be mother-in-law, would have a lengthy visit to help with the newborn. Mother has let it be known that Janet could have any man, one without canes and slurred speech. Mother has let it be known that with me, Janet was bringing her work home. Mother believes Janet only lives with me out of pity. Mother can't seem to have an unexpressed thought! Add to these stressors, the fact that I'm up for tenure and it will either be granted or I will be given a terminal contract. I'll either have a job for life or be unemployed. Announcing that she didn't want to fill a prescription is a pretty mean thing to say, especially an hour before my lecture. Too bad the Americans With Disabilities Act didn't cover this.

So after this bomb was dropped in my lap, so to speak, I managed to get to the lecture hall. Plop-slide, plop-slide, plop-slide. Today, there were no grateful librarians or children to rescue from terrorists. My burden was too great. What if I were denied tenure, terminated and penniless, with an expensive, mother-in-law filled apartment and a new mouth to feed? Maybe now is not the right time. It's not that I'm a pessimist; it's just that I'm a realist. Maybe now is not the right time.

With my mind as far from Chaucer as England is from the United States, I tried to teach about metaphors, similes and personification. Lecturing is different for a gimp professor than for one with normal limbs and speech. A normal professor can wander his or her ideas, misspeak, and lose trains of thought. It happens to normal professors all of the time. But when you have crutches and distorted speech, those normal byproducts of thought can cause rumors of mental incompetence, which obviously goes hand-in-hand with cerebral palsy. Students begin wondering if the good professor has bad thinking, and impaired thinking is a death blow for professors. Students don't like paying tuition to hear the ramblings of the retarded or demented. So, I tried hard to keep my mind on the subject at hand, periodically reviewing my woes in my mind. I finally got into a rhythm and managed to stimulate a lively, if not completely relevant, discussion. One student with a bright tattoo of an American flag surrounding a Saturday night special on his shoulder took issue with another student's comment about the Bible and personification. She was one of the new breed of students I have seen gracing the campus during the past few years. I call them Bohemians and the only thing lacking is Paris of the 1930's, the Left Bank of La Seine, and Hemingway. They hang around coffee shops, smoke cigarettes, and wear berets. They rage against the machine. She remarked that religion personifies the universe, gives humanness, and even worse, maleness, to things not human. God is a man, he had a son, there is communication in the form of prayer, yada, yada, yada. She certainly grasped the essence of personification, but also the ire of the Christians in the class. I let them argue and debate as I silently pondered responsibilities and my frail shoulders to support them. Finally, the hand of the clock crept to dismissal time and I was able to bring an end to the class. As I plop-slid toward the door, the Bohemian approached me. She muttered something about how I should be more directive in class and keep the narrow-minded from wasting time of the good minds. She said she felt uncomfortable in my class.

"Why are the broad minded suddenly so narrow minded about my time management?" Realizing I had actually said that aloud to the Bohemian, I immediately began to qualify the unintended remark. The Bohemian looked startled at first, but picked up the verbal gauntlet. She said something about feeling intimidated and began to whine that the faithful Christians' ideas distressed her good senses. She started down the victim road, professing how life, daddy, and society had done her wrong, wailing on and on about injustices, capitalism, and oppression. My back began to hurt. I can't stand too long in one place without getting these sharp pains in my back. I looked around for a place to sit. It appeared that this one-sided discussion was going to continue.

We were alone in the isle of the classroom. I realized I had never really looked at her, and until now, she was just another beret-wearing face in the class. She was in her early twenties and actually quite attractive. She had full lips, reddish-brown hair, and eyes tinted by greenish contact lenses. She dressed in black. She also had a superior, self-righteous air about her. The Bohemian's speech was punctuated with all of the politically correct buzz words. I listened intently to her, not because I wanted to, but because I couldn't get a word in edgewise. I tried to defend my time management, but she interrupted and corrected me. Apparently, I have a lot to learn about the evils of the world. And then, it came out of my untenured mouth. It simply sprang from my mouth and I was helpless to stop it. I said she had a constipation problem and she appeared bloated. Oh, heck, I actually said she was full of shit. My back was hurting, Janet's prescription was on my mind, my crutches were cutting into my wrists, and I was blocked from escaping her talk-show diatribe. It just came out. Well, that energized her. She promptly notified me that my time-management, oppression, and callousness would be reported to the Dean and several of the hordes of committees established to protect her from being uncomfortable. She let me know that she had been empowered since Head Start and that I'd pay for "dissin'" her. Then, finally, she stormed out of the classroom, and I felt relief. Had I known that was all I needed to rid her from my life, I would have said it sooner. I felt like shouting that the toilet was down the hall and to the right. Whew.

As I plop-slid back to my office, I realized I had created yet another problem to add to the mounting list. Now I would have to deal with feminists and other hate groups set on ridding the world of evil. Committees of sensitive, Alan Alda type liberal professors would review my callousness and tisk, tisk their disdain. My views on the world would be explored and examined in excruciating detail. Oh, some of them would excuse my behavior because I am disabled. There are those on campus who embrace racism, sexism, and harassment when it is done by the right people for the good of us all. This would be awful. I'd probably be sent to a Cambodian reeducation camp to learn sensitivity. The prize of tenure would certainly be denied all because of my big, spastic mouth.

Chapter Seven

My leg hurt and I do mean hurt. And I was cold. The Cessna in the stream was barely recognizable. I had the ironic thought that with two more payments, the crumpled mess would be all mine. But we were alive, more or less, and I had to think about getting us home and getting medical care. Oh God, the pain in my leg was unbearable, and I was losing blood. I got sick to my stomach when I saw the white bone protruding from above my knee, and I started to get light-headed. I saw the four of them and realized we may not have survived the crash after all. Four retards, miles from help, stranded in the outback of Alaska. My only consolation was that I had done my best, and that comforted me.

Trevor carried Nicole to a grassy clearing where sunlight cast long shadows. He laid her down gently on the pine needles serving as a mat. She was crying, wet, and cold, but she was alive. Trevor shivered both from fear and cold. Trevor's left hand had a puncture wound, but it stopped bleeding. Elroy had a nasty cut on his back and shoulder; the blood had stained his wet shirt a pinkish hue. He also felt his right side and knew something was broken. It hurt when he breathed. Rusty stood next to a large boulder, looking at the bright yellow airplane occasionally rolling and sliding down the stream, uttering: "Mayde," "Mayde," "Mayde."

Four souls with a combined IQ under 300 looked at where fate had deposited them. From the vantage point of the nearby pine trees they sat, either crying or quiet, with Elroy shaking the shoulder of the unconscious pilot, saying: "Wake-up Mr. Pilot," "Wake-up, Please." Nicole sobbed as Trevor, kneeling next to her, held her hand, trying to process the frightening events. Rusty used his fingers to strobe the sunlight, barely detectable over the surrounding mountains, and he began to rock back and forth. From the canyon ridge above the Dolores River, five humans sat or lay quietly while the yellow wreckage of the airplane bobbed and slid in the roaring, picturesque river. From the top of the mountains paralleling the canyon, only several blurry dots were visible, nothing really distinguishing them from the surroundings. From the distant view of a commercial airliner shooting across the Alaskan sky and trailing white, dissipating vapor, nothing of the crashed flying machine or frightened souls could be seen. And from the global view of communication satellites, where the long Alaskan and Canadian coastline stretched for thousands of miles, islands and glaciers could be distinguished, but there was nothing to signal the plight of the five survivors, nothing but rugged wilderness, wild, hungry animals, and the life-and-death drama that was to unfold.

Chapter Eight

Janet knew things were not going well between her and Ben. It had been weeks since their busy schedules had allowed any form of intimacy. She hoped it was their busy schedules, but in the back of her mind she feared he was avoiding her sexually. Each night, he was either already asleep when she came to bed or stayed up late to read papers, often sleeping on the old green and brown couch until daybreak. She knew he was troubled about work. He told her of some verbal altercation with one of his students. As she increased her jogging pace, she began to wonder where all of these stressors were going to take them. She felt out of control. It worried her.

It was unusually warm and she was already sweating. Birds were chirping, and in the distance she could hear the early risers speeding down State Street. She could feel her heart pounding in her chest, her hair bouncing, and tightness in her knees. It wasn't pain, just tightness, and she put more spring in her run. Jogging has so many benefits. It is healing to the mind and soul, a form of meditation. It opens pores and blood vessels. The lungs breathe deeply and the heart grows stronger. Leg and hip muscles strengthen and become firm. The morning jogger greets the day robustly and with energy. But jogging jars the hips and knees. It takes a toll on joints, but it is a small price to pay. Janet was committed to jogging. She knew she would eventually be one of those little old ladies jogging, walking really, early in the mornings in some retirement community in the South.

When she returned to their apartment, Ben had already gone to work. What possible business did he have at the University at 7:30 a.m.? He had made the coffee and left the newspaper carefully folded at her end of the table. Janet showered and dried her hair, and as she closed the door to their apartment, she realized it had become far too quiet. Janet and Ben had begun to co-exist.

It came out of the blue. There was no warning, no indication as Ron struck her hard in the face, knocking her to the ground. Janet had been teaching him the finer points of sorting recyclable paper, how colored paper went in the blue drum and all others in the yellow one, when it happened. They were alone in the large, brightly lit supply room, the door partially open. It never occurred to Janet that Ron would strike her, let alone drop to his knees, place his hands around her throat and try to choke the life from her. But he was determined to kill. With her strong running legs, she kicked at his groin, but her foot missed the sensitive target. She tried to turn on her stomach and then knock him backward, but he was too strong and too determined. She tried to scream, but his hands stopped the flow of air carrying the cry for help. In the corner of her eyes, she saw Rusty peeking through the partially opened door. He was staring at the violence, captivated by it, but too frightened and confused to help. She knew he would be a nonverbal witness to her murder. She kept fighting and struggling and then began to weaken.

Elroy usually never let Janet out of his sight when she was at the Center. But he and a supervisor had driven the Center's truck to a grocery store to pick up donated bread, buns, cookies, and cakes for the "Day Old" store. Day old? Yeah, right. Even the residents at the Center knew the foodstuffs in the store were older than a day. Elroy loved that part of his job at the Center. He got to ride in the big truck, high above the other traffic. He always purchased a soda from the grocery store after the work of loading was done. On the ride back to the Center, he'd bum a smoke from the driver, and was just learning how to inhale without coughing. He knew he was the envy of everyone watching him riding shotgun in that large truck. Ah, it was a wonderful life. He loved trips to the grocery stores.

As the truck backed into the loading dock with the beep, beep, beep warning all to run for cover, Elroy looked around for Janet. He knew she would be lonesome for him, sad and dreaming of his return. She probably spent the past hour searching the center for him. But, she was nowhere to be found. After the truck stopped and the engine turned off, Elroy began searching for her. As he walked by a door, he saw Rusty with his back to the wall, strobing and muttering: "Dodear, Dodear." Elroy thought that was strange even for Rusty.

When he opened the door, he couldn't believe his eyes. Bad Ron was hurting Janet. All of Elroy's life, he had been taught never to be violent, never to strike or hurt anyone . . . never. And Elroy fostered ill will toward no one. He loved people, all of them, even Bad Ron. What to do? He went over to two struggling bodies and shouted, "Stop it, stop it, please." Oh, what to do? "Stop it, now." He began to dance around them, his mind blocked. Then, Elroy reached down and grabbed Bad Ron by his jacket and threw him through the air and into the wall. Slowly, Janet's screams became louder and finally staff and supervisors came to her rescue. Elroy began to cry.

Chapter Nine

I usually eat lunch at home. One of the perks of professoring is that you can come and go as you wish as long as you keep regular office hours and, of course, teach your classes. But, today the Chair of the Department wanted to talk to me. We decided to have lunch at one of the small restaurants in the International Center. The International Center is the hub of the campus and sits next to the library complex in full view of Bell Tower. The Bell Tower announces the hour and half-hour with clarion music and is the beating heart of the campus. It is a splendid addition to this beautiful campus and is surrounded by rolling hills, ancient weeping willow trees, and a concert area created out of grass, bushes, and flowers. It's just below the campus stadium, which seats nearly a hundred thousand football fans. On Football Saturday, you can hear the roar of the crowd for miles. I've had season passes since I was a student.

Bob Charles is a fine person for a guy with two first names. He's been Chair of the Department for twelve years. Twelve years is a lifetime in administration. He's seen it all come and go. Every issue has been dealt with, every contingency planned for, every conflict addressed. University politics are really cutthroat. I suppose it's because you have intelligent and educated people with a sense of self-importance. But, I swear, I've seen more maturity at the Center. Once during the weekly dreaded faculty meeting, a faculty member almost threw herself on the floor kicking and wailing because she didn't get her way. Another fellow actually stood up and stormed out of the room while hurling epithets at us. These were over course scheduling conflicts. The faculty meetings are held in the department conference room—the "viper pit," as one assistant professor now calls it.

Bob was uncharacteristically late so I decided to get something to eat. I had a class in about an hour. At this cafe, you must pass through a line, plopping food on a tray that you slide along four stainless-steel bars. I suppose it is a convenience for most people, but for me, what with two metal canes protruding from my arms, it's problematic. But I was hungry, time was short, and there were no options. So, I plop-slid to the cashier and told her of my predicament. Actually, I told her twice. I have to remember to open my mouth widely and say each sound as clearly as possible or my punishment will be "Pardon? You need kelp with that ocean spray?" She was a tiny person, but well proportioned, and I liked her matter-of-fact manner. She asked me what I wanted and where I was sitting. I paid for the food in advance, and when there was a lull in the action, she brought the tray to me. I smiled and said, "Thank you."

"I'm sorry I'm late," Bob Charles said as he arrived. "I would have been here sooner but I didn't leave early enough." Bob has that droll English humor I find confusing. I never know when to laugh, or even if I should. I told him it was no problem, and that I had started lunch without him. Ever polite, he excused himself, walked to the stack of trays and began to select the blandest of food. I heard through the grapevine that he had something irritable residing in his digestive tract and could only appease it with soft, tasteless food.

Bob took a seat next to me, a little too close for my comfort. Apparently, our conversation was to be private and intimate. He had his usual worried look on his face. He was dressed in his typical administrative uniform: blue suit, red tie, and spit-shined wingtip shoes. Bob has the kind of body not designed for suit-wearing. Every suit he owns fits poorly, like clothing on a monkey. They fit too tightly in some places and too loosely in others. Bob should wear greasy coveralls like the ones worn by mechanics. The coveralls could have his name sown on them: Bob Charles, Chair. He'd finally look comfortable.

Pity is the worst. It is by far the worst part of being disabled, and Bob occasionally teeters over the line separating it from compassion. Pity belittles me while providing an ego boost for the ones dispensing it. Fortunately, I knew Bob's purpose when he teetered toward pity. It was to help me and to make my life a little easier. Bob was as close to a friend as I had in the Department.

As he began to eat the non-irritating sandwich and slurp his bland soup, he announced: "You are in trouble with the Promotion and Tenure Committee." Between bites, he explained that my student evaluations, while good, were not in the upper quartile for the Department and several students said I was hard to understand. And although I had published two novels, several articles in literary journals, and one in a national weekly magazine, the quality of my scholarship was "borderline." "Publish or perish," he said. Adding to the litany of bad news, he said I was also being investigated for the heinous crime of insensitivity. Apparently, the Bohemian had followed through on her threat. Bob put his hand on my shoulder and said, "We'll get through this. You know you have my support, but it'll be a battle."

And then Bob made me angry. In so many roundabout words, he said I should play the "disabled card." I should use it as a preemptive strike. I should go to one of the committees charged with making college comfortable and say I was being bullied *because of my disabilities.* I should become the victim.

Once again, my spastic mouth took over and I reactively told him: "Sure, Bob, I'll also buy a beret, take up smoking, and start wearing black." He didn't have a clue what that meant, and I didn't feel the need to explain. I was pissed.

I have had conflicts with several of the Promotion and Tenure Committee members. One member, a woman who reminded me of "Mother," had complained I teach too much "White, European Male" literature. Other committee members were simply jealous of my novels. Two commented I pandered to the pathetic populace. They condemned the books because the great unwashed masses actually bought and read them. One of the comments on my peer review said I lacked "collegiality." That's professor-speak for not being right-minded. People expect me to be ever so politically correct, liberal on politics, antiguns, antismoking, anti this, that, and the other thing, and vocal for massive government programs to rescue the downtrodden. I'm not, never have been, and never will be, and it upsets people. Too bad. Deal with it. Oh, the viper pit was active during my tenure deliberations.

Bob was right. I was in trouble with the Committee, but it wasn't because of my cerebral palsy, slurred speech, raspy voice, and gimpness. It was because they disapproved of my performance. They simply disliked me for being me. You gotta love people like that. I was disliked and disapproved of for all of the right reasons, the same ones that had caused three professors in the past year to be denied promotion and tenure. It was the same petty crap, and I admired them for it. No way would I play the disabled card. Let the cards fall where they may. Some things are more important than promotion and tenure. Some things are more important than job security. Some things are more important than happiness.

About the time I finished explaining to Bob my reasons for not playing the disabled card, my cell phone rang. It was a social worker at the hospital telling me Janet had been admitted. She quickly told me Janet was in good condition and she was just being held for observation. Then my heart stopped racing and my hands shaking, I told Bob of the family emergency and went to the hospital. I met the social worker in the lobby and together we went to Janet's room. I couldn't believe my eyes.

Janet was asleep. A nurse said she had been sedated. She laid between the crisp, white hospital sheets with her long, dark hair flowing over a small pillow; Sleeping Beauty with a huge black, red, and blue eye. There were stitches running from her eyebrow. When I saw the bluish finger marks around her long, sensual neck, I got sick to my stomach and felt the need to go to the bathroom. For an instant, I thought I'd caught something irritable from Bob. I felt tears run down my face and I went to the window and looked at the busy parking lot. Oddly, I felt both joy and rage. I wanted to hug Janet, tell her I loved her and then drive to the Center and kill Bad Ron: that son-of-a-bitch.

Janet never talked about it, to me anyway. After she was discharged from the hospital, I took her home and did my best to nurse her psychologically and physically. I catered to her every need. She read and did needlepoint. She slept late into the mornings, which was unusual. For two weeks, she cleaned the apartment, polished our sparse silverware, talked on the phone to "Mother," and did laundry. She asked about my work, cared for me, and kept busy. Every time I broached the subject, thinking it would be good for her to talk about it, she politely refused. On the Sunday morning before she returned to work, while we ate bagels in bed and read the Sunday *Journal,* I again tried to get her to talk about it. No way. I realized that for Janet, the subject was closed. Some things are too private, too personal, and we would never discuss it. If that was how she was going to deal with her attempted murder, then so be it. Whatever it takes. Monday morning, Janet awoke early, donned her jogging clothes, and resumed her life. Bad Ron was history. I did note that around her neck hung a small silver whistle and gray tube of extra-strength pepper spray. That afternoon, I went to Big Jake's Guns and Liquor and signed a document promising I wasn't insane or criminal. I bought a .22-caliber semiautomatic pistol and placed it in the small drawer next to my side of the bed. For Janet, Bad Ron may be history, but he had taken my security and the gun helped restore it. $395.00 is a small price to pay for a sense of security.

Chapter Ten

Finals week drew a bad semester to a close. Faculty are required to attend every other graduation ceremony, but I attend them all. I love the pomp and circumstance, the marching, the gowns, and the elated students with conferred degrees. I listen to the speaker's talk of lofty goals and sadly noting the end of an important part of life. Caps are thrown in the air, students and parents cry, and faculty are hugged. It is a time of beginnings and endings. For me, I feared it was more ending than beginning. The Promotion and Tenure Committee had sent their secretive report to the Dean and Provost. I would be notified of their decision after our return from Alaska. Apparently, there was some delay with my application. I hate the waiting. I was getting a little edgy.

I was avoiding the issue of children and unfilled prescriptions like the plague. Maybe the time wasn't right for another mouth to feed. For three weeks, Janet and I simply caught glimpses of each other going through doors, driving out of the apartment complex, eating sandwiches, and falling to sleep. For the first week after Janet returned to work, sex was out of the question. I knew the daily birth control pills had run out and danger lurked in the bedroom. I could rid sex from my life. Monks, priests, and nerds did it all of the time. No man ever died from a lack of sex. I could do celibacy standing on my head. I breezed through the first week. During the second week, I continued to avoid Janet and bed, though I did find myself watching her walk and talk with more interest. She has soft hands. The nape of her neck is as sensual as her smell. I love the curve of her body as she lies on the couch, particularly where waist meets hip. Janet also wears reading glasses; need I say more? One morning, I found myself studying newspaper ads for bras and panties. Those models were certainly shameless. I recalled from my youth nasty pictures in Playboy of wanton women wearing about the same amount of clothing as seen in those ads, which today boldly take up an entire page of a newspaper. At work, I found it difficult to maintain eye-contact with busty women. By the third week, a millennium without sex, I began rethinking my position on children. Like I said, I was getting a little edgy. So, like a remorseful puppy, one night I left the stack of term papers, slipped into bed with Janet, and began caressing her, my pathetic nonverbal way of initiating. She met me with open, unprotected arms. What the heck, maybe the time was right for children. Let's cross that bridge later. Afterward, I felt pretty good about my resolve. Three weeks of sexual self-denial. Not bad. Janet slept smugly, all along knowing how this would work out. I slept an entire night for the first time in three weeks and awoke the next morning refreshed and renewed, but knowing one thing for certain: I am a weak man. Like my cerebral palsy, it's just another part of my life to accept. I took solace in the fact that most men are sexual cripples.

The night before we were to leave for Anchorage, the Center was abuzz with excitement. Rusty was constantly strobing, rocking and uttering "cheska," a reference to something no one could decipher. We had given him a map with yellow markings showing our path from Anchorage to Fairbanks, and then to the wilderness cabin. He kept pointing to it saying, "cheska." Elroy wanted to share a suitcase with Janet and trailed her from room to room. He always managed to be standing between me and Janet, with his back to me. He's a cocky one, all right. Anastasia locked herself in her bedroom and we had to get a master key to console her. Nicole and Trevor packed together, talking about necessary items. Janet had to remove half of what they packed and replace it with items a little more practical for an Alaskan adventure. For some reason, Trevor believed shoe polish and a small reading lamp would be necessary. I could almost understand the shoe polish, but reading was not one of Trevor's strengths. Nicole carefully placed her birth control pills in the small carrying case full of toiletries. Janet and Melissa had taught her the intricacies of Planned Parenthood. The next day at 6:50 a.m. we would begin our great adventure. Late that evening, Janet and I returned home and once again, I set my swimmers free to find her elusive egg. I was beginning to like the idea of being a father. I was a lot more relaxed.

I had met with the "Committee" charged with reviewing my conduct with the Bohemian, and it wasn't as awful as I thought it would be. I expected a committee of spineless wonders, strapped to their chairs so they wouldn't tumble to the floor. But they patiently listened to the Bohemian and then gave me my turn. She went on and on about her comfort level and how I had probably ruined her life, a job begun by her daddy and our founding fathers. The pain she felt was incredible. When it was my turn, I simply held my ground. There would be no remorse and no undoing. As far as I was concerned, I had a God-given right to say anything and everything I felt was important. Notice that I said God-given right. You see, I don't have much physical freedom what with canes and spastic muscles. Consequently, freedom of speech is very important to me. I don't believe the government, or anyone else for that matter, has the right to control someone's speech. Period, and it's not open for discussion. How's that for a contradiction? Freedom of speech is too important to me, society, evolution, and life. And a lot of soldiers have died face down in the mud to protect it. I'll say what's on my mind and if the powers that be don't like it, too bad. Arrest me, fire me, execute me. I'll say what's on my mind and damn the consequences. I'll also run my courses the way I see fit. I believe in academic freedom. As I told the "Committee," let the Bohemian get several degrees, teach for nearly a decade, age for two more, and then I might be interested in her myopic opinions of my course management. I then told the "Committee" of her constipation and bloating problem.

I was surprised that many on the committee shared my views. Oh, there were several who talked of limits of freedom. I let them talk and even listened, though I've heard it before. I didn't feel unbearable discomfort at what they had to say, even though I couldn't have disagreed more. Finally, the committee reached a decision that there would be no censure or reprimand. One member commented to the Bohemian that if other people's ideas made her so uncomfortable, maybe she was not ready for college; maybe she needed a little time off for introspection. At the conclusion of the meeting, I felt elated. The Bohemian stormed from the Faculty Senate Hearing Room convinced of yet more oppression, and I knew she would continue to rage against the machine. Life goes on. In my office later that evening, I sent an E-mail to the Bohemian. I apologized for my insensitivity.

Chapter Eleven

Someone wrapped my leg with a tattered shirt. The pain diminished to a constant throb accompanied by a burning sensation. I was still light-headed, but alive. I knew that below the blood-soaked tattered shirt, the bone of my leg was still protruding from the skin. Curiously, I thought of how the makeshift bandage would protect my body from invasion of ants and bloodsucking maggots. My life-savior was shaking my shoulder demanding I awaken. I pushed his hand aside, and slowly, painfully, slid myself into a half-sitting position with my back to a boulder. He stopped talking and awaited my leadership. I realized that unless my distress call was heard by other pilots, my instructions were going to be simple: "Prepare to kiss your butts goodbye."

The sun was setting. Well, at this time of year in Alaska, it really doesn't set. It just gets lower in the sky. But it was dark because of the trees, canyon and mountains. I was cold and I knew we needed a fire. A fire would provide warmth and also a beacon for search planes. I told my savior to get kindling and wood together, and I would somehow muster the strength to use my lighter to get a fire started. He and the one called "Trevor," quickly rose to the occasion and soon had enough down and dead wood for a warming beacon. Dead grass and moss crumpled under the kindling and soon burst into flame as fire was released. Another irony. I was happy my attempts to quit smoking were unsuccessful, and put the prized lighter back in my pocket. I told the passengers to keep the fire burning. I said it loudly and several times. They're retarded after all. Again, I passed out.

Rusty, Nicole, Trevor, and Elroy moved close to the small fire. It warmed them physically and psychologically. Soon, everyone had fallen asleep, not so much from fatigue, but as a temporary escape from the fear. The crackling of the fire and deep breathing was drowned in the roar of the Dolores River. Soon, the fire died as the passengers slept. Hours later, Elroy awoke. He again shook the shoulder of the pilot, but there was no response. He looked around. Nicole and Trevor slept in each other's arms. Rusty was awake, but he just stared at the smoke rising from the dead fire. Elroy thought of Janet and knew she must be worried about him. He was cold and his side felt like a spear had penetrated it. Elroy knew he must find her. Forgetting the "Hug a Tree" lecture, he stood up, left the camp and began the search for Janet and the rescue party he knew she would be leading. Rusty continued to stare at the smoke rising from the dead fire. Nicole, without opening her eyes, pulled Trevor closer, and they shared lifesaving body heat.

Nyle was from Liverpool, but had lived and worked in Alaska for twenty-four years. His only regret was that in Alaska, women are rare. It's about five to one in most towns and cities, and in real Alaska, the vast wilderness, it was more like a hundred to one for unattached females. After a quarter of a century, he was still searching for the woman to share his life. But, Nyle was already in love. His first and only love was flying, and being a bush pilot in Alaska was a dream come true. Each day was a scenic adventure. Today, he was taking a young couple to Tuktoyuktuk for a hiking and camping honeymoon when he heard the "May Day." He was short on fuel and knew an immediate response was dangerous. Two downed planes would help no one. He contacted Fairbanks Tower and told them of the emergency. They heard part of the distress call, but were unable to detect anything on radar. Air Search and Rescue was alerted and pilots from Fairbanks and surrounding areas left jobs and family to search for one of their kind.

Chapter Twelve

If you are a people watcher, like me, airports are voyeur heaven— thousands of people rushing, waiting, drinking, eating, and shuffling heavy luggage down wide corridors. After the Center's bus deposited us at the loading zone where bright red signs threatened to execute us if, even for a second, there was loitering, we became part of the human mass swelling to gates and airplanes. After our luggage was placed on conveyor belts and sped off to parts unknown, we began the long journey to Gate 17 in Terminal Three.

I don't know whether normal people are stared at during these journeys, but we were the objects of people's attention. Now I know how famous rock groups feel when they embark and disembark airplanes. I suppose we did look a sight. Janet, lead singer and female sex object, took the lead and set the pace followed by Drummer Rusty strobing and occasionally uttering "cheska." I brought up the rear, following the rhythm section: Anastasia, Trevor and Nicole. Our pace was slow, but we had plenty of time. If normals must be at the airport one hour before takeoff, we knew to double the lead time. We politely refused the offer to ride on one of the golf carts to be rushed to the gate. That seemed like cheating. Let our great adventure begin in this airport and the lessons of independence and character start with the long hike to the first of three airplanes. As we made our way most people stared, but they keep going. Some actually stopped just to observe us. Two children shouted, "Look Daddy." Twice, I stopped and returned their stares and once, just for the fun of it, I strobed like Rusty.

Over the years, I have learned that airport travelers are not being rude or mean at their unbroken eye-contact. It's unconscious on their part. They just see something unusual, and it takes time for them to process it. They're like Trevor. It takes time to figure out what the heck is going on. They wonder about our destination, purpose, and means. They wonder who is retarded and who in charge. On a deeper level, they ponder the meaning of life. Why are we the way we are and they spared our plight? Oh, some are distressed that we exist and are angry that we don't know our place. Aren't there institutions for our kind? Doesn't government have places where we are cared for by well-spent tax dollars? Twice, I have heard drunks at airports make unkind jokes. Of course, they're crippled by alcohol, a fear of flying, and a tendency to shout nonsense.

I watch them, too. I see families off to reunions, divorced dads sending children back to their "biological" mothers, grandparents headed to winter retreats, and students returning to their studies. There are business travelers with plans of hostile takeovers. The most interesting of travelers are the lovers rejoicing or despairing. They hug and share long kisses. They stroke arms and backs waiting for the painful separation. They squeal and embrace with smiles so permanent they will need to be surgically removed. It is a drama watching people at airports, and we appeared to be the main act. I plop-slide onto one of the moving sidewalks. My canes leave far too quickly for my reluctant feet, and for an instant, I'm stretched like an elastic band. Trevor and Nicole appear to enjoy the people mover the most. It's like a ride at Disneyland, but without the long lines. They share puppy dog looks of intimacies and secrets only young lovers know. There is a glow about them.

We finally reach the gate and begin the long wait before we can speed through the thin atmosphere. Hurry up and wait. I stack my canes on the next plastic seat and continue the theater. Just who would be sharing the first leg of our adventure with us? It seems there will be the usual composition: old, young, colored, uncolored, tall, short, loud, soft, business, and recreational. It will be a diverse group of sardines in the tin. I take comfort in seeing the babies and toddlers. I know God and pilots would never let the plane crash with such precious cargo. Uh-oh: Nicole and Trevor are holding hands and looking deeply into each other's eyes as they talk of their world. I'm envious of the magic they share, but I look to see if there are ugly people on our adventure. Young love among the physically and mentally disabled sometimes brings out the worst in people. But if facial expressions show what people are thinking, then our compatriots on this journey are not distressed. We are with the live-and-let-live crowd.

Finally, the attendant announces those passengers crippled by success, spastic muscles, and small children can board first. Ordinarily, I board with the rest of the sardines, refusing to play the disabled card. But because of my companions, this time I play the game. As I give my boarding pass to the uniformed attendant, he announces that our party will experience "first class." Apparently, on this flight there was a shortage of the rich and the airline, knowing our defects, bumped us to the elite. We would have more room for crutches, seizures, strobing, drooling, and stretching out on the long flight to

Anchorage. We would also have hot facial towels (I make a mental note to see how Rusty handles hot towels), unlimited beverages, and attention. We would have two choices of meals and all the peanuts that could be digested. We boarded first and were the envy of all others shuffling down the aisle to their second-class status.

The flight to Anchorage was long and unremarkable. I sat by Janet only after convincing Elroy that the audio headset worked best in a window seat. The airplane was one of the jumbo jets, a DC something or other. We were pampered by the flight attendant and watched an old Disney movie about dogs and cats trying to return home. Rusty strobed and rocked during the entire flight, much to the irritation of the passenger setting behind him. Anastasia slept some of the flight or simply reclined in her seat with her eyes closed. Twice she took Rusty's strobing hand and forced it in his lap. Rusty was also getting on Anastasia's nerves. Nicole and Trevor sat together in the seats closest to the curtain separating us from the second class riffraff. I don't think they stopped holding hands even during the meal. The flight was smooth and comfortable, but most of the time, the clouds below us blocked the view. I read, slept, and ate enough peanuts to fill a small elephant. Janet spent more time in the restroom than all of us. Flying makes her airsick.

Across the aisle was another first classer sitting next to her husband. She was one of those direct people who simply asked about us. She was curious. I told her of the Center and the grant. She asked very intelligent questions about Rusty, Anastasia and me. We struck up an easy, temporary friendship. I wondered if the quality of conversation was as good in second class.

Chapter Thirteen

Nyle made a perfect three-point landing. The Piper Cub, a tail-dragger, touched down lightly and simultaneously on all three wheels. Soon, a large truck with two grades of fuel paralleled his airplane. Within twenty minutes, the Piper's wing tanks were full. Nyle grabbed a sandwich and coffee from the vending machine, went to the bathroom, and was in the cockpit in time to sign for the fuel. He decided to forego the preflight check, got tower clearance, and soon was racing to the Dolores River. The nighttime sun, dim and barely perceptible over the horizon, provided enough light for six hours of searching. He determined to drop below the canyon and simply follow the Dolores River to the inlet. Flying low and fast through a canyon was dangerous, but the sense of speed was exhilarating. Only good pilots dared do it, and Nyle was a good pilot. At 120 knots he sped through the Dolores Canyon, the roar of the propeller and engine frightening several fishing grizzlies. They ran in search of safety from the huge bird of prey. He hoped he wouldn't meet some other search plane coming in the opposite direction.

I awoke again, my leg throbbing and my head pounding with pain. I saw the fire had died. I shouted for Elroy and Trevor. Trevor came to me but there was no sign of Elroy. I asked Trevor where Elroy was, and after a brief delay, he said: "Janet. He find Janet." My stomach turned to a knot, and I knew there would be the report of at least one fatality. Damn it. I thought of sending Trevor to find him, but I knew he would also get lost, and that would lead to two reports of fatalities. I shouted for Elroy to return to the safety of the camp, but there was no response. The Dolores River was too loud and I was too weak. With Trevor's help, we again achieved fire. I hoped Elroy was not too far away to see the smoke. I wondered if he would have the brains to return to camp. I slipped into unconsciousness, certain their frightened faces would be my last image of this world.

After thirty minutes of walking, Elroy was hopelessly lost. He could see nothing familiar, and even the sound of the river was gone. He was frightened and cold. Elroy could think of nothing but Janet as he began to run in the direction he knew would lead to their reunion. He ran for nearly an hour through trees and bushes before he collapsed on a big, smooth rock. He started to cry. Then, in the distance, he heard a low-pitched growl. Frightened at the sound of what he knew was a hungry bear the size of a truck, Elroy again ran. He ran and ran and ran. Finally, he sat with his back to a large pine tree.

About an hour from Tucktoyuktuk, Nyle saw smoke spiraling from the canyon. Knowing that slow, low and heavy was dangerous for any airplane, he climbed above the canyon and circled it. He made three low, but fast passes over the source of the smoke. Each time he saw the yellow wreckage of the airplane and several people. He continued to circle above the crash site while he radioed Fairbanks. A search and rescue helicopter was diverted to his location, and soon was setting down at a small clearing just above a bend in the river. He saw the rescuers rush to the downed airplane and the frightened passengers. They waved and announced they had the rescue under control. Nyle then pushed the throttle forward on his Piper and began a gradual upward spiral to clear the high canyon walls. He dipped wings several time in farewell, and began the flight home. On the forest floor, Elroy looked up, wiped his tears, and saw the airplane shoot across the sky.

Chapter Fourteen

Janet had thrown up three mornings in a row. Locked in the small restroom of the airplane, she tried to kneel in such a way as to contain it. The good news was that there was nothing to empty from her stomach. The better news was that she was pregnant. The bad news was that she was pregnant *now.* As she flushed the vacuum driven toilet, she thought that perhaps Ben was right. Maybe now was not the right time. Janet had miscalculated. Apparently, it is a lot easier to get pregnant than she had thought. After reaching her seat, Janet watched Anchorage approach through the small portal. She was surprised at how large the city was.

The huge jet, a "heavy" as it is called by the tower, touched down as smooth and gentle as a seagull. Janet helped the adventurers disembark. After collecting themselves, they walked and shuffled to a small cafe. They feasted on very expensive sandwiches, slices of pizza, hamburgers, and colas. Watching them eat, Janet thought how fortunate she was to be able to share this time with them. So many people in the world are unremarkable. They strive to wear the same clothes, express the same sentiments, and to live ordinary, mundane lives. In the world of people, most are like bland vanilla ice cream in a store offering thirty-one flavors. But not her people. They entered this world different and unique. Her people viewed and responded to the world on their own terms and in their own exceptional ways. They had innocence uncontaminated by mediocrity.

Rusty sat on the edge of his chair chewing mouthful after mouthful of potato salad. He was completely caught up in the sight, texture, smell, and taste of it. Janet could tell that for Rusty, nothing else in the world existed but the yellow food; his world *was* potato salad. Anastasia picked at her pizza slice. She had carefully removed the pastrami, olives, peppers, and chunks of sausage. Between bites, she cautiously scanned the dining room looking for threats of danger. Her mother's drinking problem caused Anastasia to be fearful of strangers. Janet chuckled silently to herself as she saw Nicole and Trevor arguing about napkins and straws. Apparently, someone neglected to place them on their tray. Were clouds brewing in paradise? Would too much closeness cause a spat? Elroy sat next to Janet eating nearly $20.00 worth of airport food. Janet had to remind him to slow down. He had a tendency to gulp an entire meal. Janet lacked elbow room because, as usual, Elroy sat too close to her. And then there was Ben, the father of her unborn child. He sat quietly, slowly picking at a hamburger and fries, lost in thought.

Boarding the smaller jet was quick and easy even though they had to suffer the indignities of second class. It was a short flight, in Alaska terms, to Fairbanks. As decoration, the airport in Fairbanks had stuffed Arctic animals in glass containers. Most New York museums would be envious of the collection. Everything from polar bears to eagles graced the wide corridors. The adventurers were mesmerized by the bears. Elroy starred at their sharp, white teeth and wondered how many smaller animals had been ripped and torn by them. Bears frightened him. Two taxis transported the adventurers to the Great Alaskan Hotel for needed sleep. The boys shared a room and the girls bunked together. Exhausted, they slept for nearly ten hours.

The next morning, they returned to the Fairbanks airport and met with the bush pilot who would ferry them to the cabin. His airplane sat six, and it was decided Janet and Anastasia would fly first to the wilderness cabin along with some of the provisions. They would have roughly two hours to ready it before the next flight arrived consisting of Rusty, Trevor, Nicole, and Elroy. Ben would follow on the final flight along with the rest of the supplies. It would take most of the day for the party and provisions to be transported to the cabin.

The bush pilot was obviously uncomfortable around physically and mentally impaired people. He was polite enough. He greeted us with a broad smile and shook our hands, except Rusty's. When he talked to everyone except Janet, he spoke slowly and loudly. He was in his early forties, short and stocky. It appeared flying had caused premature aging, because his hair was almost completely gray. He sported a gray moustache and expensive pilot's glasses. He wore a baseball-type cap which had "Winslow Ground Service" printed on it. The single-engine airplane, obviously his pride and joy, was bright yellow. He loaded some of the supplies in the back seat and inside luggage compartment, and other smaller boxes and duffel bags in an outside cranny. He explained to Janet that the airplane had to be balanced or takeoff would be compromised. After loading was done, he helped Anastasia in the back seat, and fastened her seat and shoulder belts. Then, he helped Janet into the front passenger seat and carefully snapped her seat and shoulder belts. I felt like clubbing him with one of my metal canes.

I knew Janet must be the most attractive woman he had ever secured in that yellow airplane. I could tell he was awestruck with her beauty and manner, and he put on quite a show, strutting for her benefit. Flyboy was hitting on her: "Oh, look at me. I can fly an airplane." I've seen it all before, but it's still hard to deal with. I'm standing there with canes and spastic speech muscles, while the devil-may-care Flyboy is preparing to make my woman soar. Oh, it's sexual all right. Jealousy saturated my thoughts and I nearly panicked. What if Janet finally reached her senses and fell hopelessly in love with Flyboy, moved permanently to Alaska, never visited a pharmacy, and had twelve little Flyboys all sporting expensive sunglasses? I would be dumped by the only love of my pathetic, cerebral-palsied life. I finally cooled down and realized that my insecurities were rearing their ugly heads. My brain again controlled my emotions. Love is blind faith, and I had to believe that Janet would remain mine. I had to believe she saw through my rivals and never gave them a second thought. I had to believe Janet was real and not some female aberration. I had to believe Janet had a blind spot. I waved to them as the airplane sped past us and slowly climbed into the great Alaskan sky. We walked back to the small coffee shop and awaited Flyboy's return.

Chapter Fifteen

The female grizzly bear had only been awake from her hibernation coma a few weeks. During the cold winter months, she had given birth to two cubs. They were constantly hungry and full of energy. After leaving the small cave, they began to descend the mountain, looking for food. The playful cubs frolicked and tumbled down hill after hill while the female grizzly hunted. They finally reached a small tributary of the Dolores River and feasted on fish. The female grizzly began the task of teaching the cubs how to hunt and fare for themselves. The huge bear sprung onto her back legs and thrust her nose into the air, sniffing for prey. The cubs imitated the behavior but tumbled over. Early one evening, she detected a vaguely familiar smell, one she had experienced years ago at the Williams City Dump. It was the scent of a human.

Chapter Sixteen

Janet hoped she wouldn't need the milk carton. Apparently, in smaller airplanes milk cartons served as barf bags. Her pilot said they also served as urinals on long flights where landing for a pit stop was out of the question. So far, so good, she thought. Her stomach and bladder were willing to contain their contents, at least for the moment. Besides, she doubted she could hit the container given the bumpy ride. A small airplane, and this one appeared to be the smallest of the small, bounced around like an old jalopy on a rocky road. She also thought the plane needed a muffler or something. One would certainly go deaf without the head set muffling the noise. She looked behind her and saw Anastasia with terror on her face. She reached for her hand, but it was pulled away. Anastasia did not want to be comforted. The pilot had a big grin on his face as he made the necessary adjustment to keep the airplane aloft. He kept talking above the noise, shouting information about destination, speed and scenic landmarks. Janet looked down at the miles of forest, rivers, mountains, and valleys, and thought how beautiful Alaska was. Below, a herd of elk or reindeer ran across a river, frightened at the sound of the noisy airplane. Janet tried to signal Anastasia to the wild beauty below, but her eyes were closed tightly and she muttered something to herself. When the pilot saw the stampeding herd, he banked the airplane sharply, lowered the nose, and shot over the herd, further scattering them. Flyboy called the maneuver a "buzz." It was a thrilling, beautiful sight.

Toward the end of the flight, Anastasia became more relaxed and even opened her eyes to the beauty below them. The rustic log cabin approached in the distance. It was larger than Janet expected and nestled in a grove of trees just above the Dolores River. There was a small dirt landing strip about two football fields from it, where the airplane would land. Flyboy said he often used water pontoons in Alaska. Lakes and rivers provided ready-made smooth landing strips. But there was no lake close to the cabin, and the Dolores River was too shallow for a water landing. The yellow airplane banked and smoothly landed on the small dirt airstrip. After the propeller ceased turning, Flyboy helped Janet and Anastasia out and they walked the short distance to the two-story cabin. A fire was started in the old wood stove, and soon the cabin was warm and toasty. It was a beautiful retreat, with golden wooden floors, couches made of logs and cushions, and large windows overlooking the river. Anastasia was captivated at the large head of a long-deceased moose overlooking the dining room. Janet and Anastasia began unpacking the supplies while they waited for grinning Flyboy and more adventurers.

Elroy was frightened and it was an overwhelming fear. The only reprieve he had from it was when he thought of Janet. Never did he entertain the thought that she was not leading a rescue in his direction, soon to embrace him with those wonderful, warm arms. Elroy was cold, shivering, and he looked around for warmth. He decided to crawl under a downed tree and hide from the cold and hungry bears. He kept thinking of the huge white teeth on the glass-enclosed airport bears. Twice, he shouted "Janet, I'm here."

In the distance, Ben saw Flyboy and his yellow airplane approach the airport. First it was just a dot on the horizon, then a larger blot, and finally a yellow blip with wings. After he landed and taxied to the flight center, Flyboy helped Elroy, Rusty, Nicole, and Trevor into the small airplane. Ben watched as they taxied to the end of the runway. He heard the engine rev, testing its strength, and then gradually gain speed until the three wheels lifted off the runway and into the Alaskan blue. He saw Nicole wave at him as the airplane dipped its wing and flew southwest toward the cabin. Ben plopped and slid back to the coffee shop to await his turn.

Janet and Anastasia waited patiently for the return of Flyboy and the rest of the crew. The two-hour wait turned into four and then six alarming hours. Patience turned to panic when a helicopter landed on the bank of the Dolores River and Ben, the pilot, and a sheriff's deputy hurried to the cabin. The bad news was confirmed by the deputy, but he assured her all that could be done was being done to find them.

They waited anxiously during of the night. Early that morning, they heard the chop, chop, chop of the helicopter and saw it land. Elation turned to angst when all disembarked but Elroy. The pilot gave little hope of finding him. Alaska can be a desolate place. Air Search and Rescue frantically continued to scan the endless wilderness for Elroy, or God forbid his body. Five airplanes, two helicopters, and three ground teams scoured a radius of fifty miles from the bobbing yellow airplane. The intense search continued for almost a week. On the sixth day, the deputy said they were going to call off the search for Elroy. They had given up hope. The weather or animals certainly had ended Elroy's life.

Chapter Seventeen

The world seems more frightening for people with high IQs. Perhaps it is because they can imagine the multitude of things that can go wrong. When the word "ignorance" is used to signify low intelligence, then bliss can go hand-in-hand with it. Certainly, Elroy didn't feel bliss, but he also didn't appreciate the gravity of his predicament. On the first day, he ran or walked over twenty miles from the crash scene. His bright red jacket would have been seen from the air had he not hidden under the dead tree. He slept there that night. On the second day, Elroy kept moving. He walked, rested, ran, rested, walked, and took shelter from the light rain under another downed tree. He was tired, hungry, and thirsty. He saw several bushes with green spring berries, but he never thought of them as edible. This was fortunate because they were poisonous. Throughout his ordeal, he had one and only one persistent thought: to find Janet.

The news that the search was being discontinued caused Janet to cry and Ben to be outraged. But the Sheriff's deputy explained in logical detail that Elroy could be anywhere in a fifty square mile area. The rescuers felt it was likely he had already fallen prey to wild animals or died from exposure. They said they had done all that could be done, and expressed their heartfelt sorrow at the loss. After they left, Ben and Janet sat solemnly at the large wooden dinner table under the watchful eyes of the long-deceased moose and talked of options. After a few minutes, they both agreed continuing the search for Elroy was the only acceptable one. They called the bush pilot who spotted the wreck and hired him to continue the search. He would charge $175.00 per hour for each of the twelve hours of search time per day. Out of their sparse savings, Ben and Janet would pay nearly two thousand dollars per day to continue the search for Elroy. When that ran out, Ben would pay the pilot from his pension. He would quit the University, draw his pension in total, pay hefty taxes and penalties, and continue the search for Elroy until it, too, ran out. After their money ran out, Ben and Janet agreed they would search on foot. Never did they entertain the idea of quitting. They would give up the search for Elroy when he was found.

Several times, the female grizzly stood on her hind legs, sniffing the air. She definitely registered the scent of a human and began the search for her prey. The wind carried the scent and she walked rapidly in the direction of its origin. The young cubs could barely keep up. She growled a hungry warning to other animals stalking the same prey. The female grizzly was no stranger to the hunt.

On the third day of the private search, Janet told Nyle to fly to the highest peak in the search radius. Trying to put herself in Elroy's place, and knowing how he thought, it occurred to her that he would go to the highest peak. Elroy was like that. He would seek the brightest and highest. His optimism would dictate his course, and Janet wondered why she had not thought of it before. Nyle said the highest peak was nearly one hundred miles from the crash scene and he doubted Elroy or anyone could have traveled that far in such a short time. But, he reluctantly agreed, and soon they were searching an 8,000 foot mountain peak with an idyllic lake nestled just below the summit.

Elroy reached the lake and drank icy cold water. He scooped the water into his hand and took gulp after gulp until satisfied. Muddy, he slid onto his side, and in a fetal position, began shaking from cold and fear. Overhead, he could hear the sound of an airplane, but he was too tired to wave or shout. In the trees bordering the lake, he heard a low-pitched growl and bushes rustling, but he was too tired to run, too tired to respond. He lay there dreaming of Janet, warmth, food and the Center.

As the small airplane flew over the lake, Janet scanned the shoreline. At first, it appeared it was simply a rock of a different color, but as she stared at it, she thought she detected movement. She pointed to it and Nyle dipped the airplane wing providing a better view. Then, she saw more movement and knew it was Elroy. Elation turned to terror when she saw a bear running from the trees toward him.

Chapter Eighteen

I hate funerals. They make me sad and they make me wonder. Unfortunately, I've attended more than my share of them. This funeral was basically the same as all of the others. I suppose that is the purpose of funerals—to be the same and to take thinking out of the process of bidding permanent farewell. Fortunately, I was spared the awful "viewing" of the body, because this one was "closed casket." I hate plop-sliding by a dead person, gazing at the body, and wondering where the spark of life had gone. I think of dead bodies as shells— containers of thought and emotion. I wonder why people call them morticians rather than the more descriptive "undertakers." I wonder if my metal crutches will be buried with me when I die.

Janet sat next to me while the speaker spoke of a life well-spent and of an untimely passing. If the quality of one's life is measured by how many people attend the funeral, then this life was well spent. The funeral was attended by hundreds of people, and many stood throughout the ritual at the back of the room. Relatives and friends spoke of family and friendship. Bitter and sweet memories were shared with all in attendance. Janet put her hand on mine as a song of remembrance was sung. Then, Elroy reached over, removed her hand from mine, and placed it firmly back in her lap. He's a cocky one, all right. When the song ended, we drove in the procession to Flyboy's final resting place. As the casket was lowered into the Alaskan ground, I wondered about life and death. Why do some people die from lost blood and others live because the sound of an airplane buzzing overhead frightens even the most determined of bears?

Chapter Nineteen

Steinbeck's *Of Mice and Men* disturbs me. It's not that Steinbeck isn't a great writer; the story disturbs me. So does the movie *Sling Blade*. They are both about murder and the mentally deficient. Ever since Bad Ron tried to kill Janet, I have been thinking about mentally deficient people and their capability for extreme good and evil. Just like the rest of us, they seem to possess tremendous good and devastating evil. In *Of Mice and Men*, Lennie Small kills because he doesn't understand his own strength. Karl Childers, in *Sling Blade*, kills because in his mind, there are no other options. What motive did Bad Ron have for attempting to take my love from me? Was it out of frustration, lack of options, or simply brain chemistry gone awry? Bad Ron is back at the Center. He is watched by staff 24-7 and wears a chemical straight-jacket. He is so medicated that violence is not an option.

What causes nobility in the mentally deficient? Where do the Elroy's of the world come from? Do loyalty, love, and courage spring from brain chemistry gone virtuous? Or, like in the rest of us, does it arise from the innate and unblocked goodness of humanity. Perhaps, goodness cannot be suppressed by the lack of synapses and cortical sugar. As I scan the bright faces of my students desperately trying to relate to mice, men, California in the 1930s, and the reasons the Pulitzer family awarded Steinbeck literary honor, I know people and motives really never change. Humans, whether they are searching for a dream ranch or simply trying to survive the desperation of an economic and spiritual depression, are capable of nobility and ignominy. Intelligence is not the variable. It all about heart, not mind.

Nearly six months have passed since our great Alaskan Adventure. In my classroom, I see the Bohemian has decided to weather yet another semester of intellectual inferiors waxing on and on about the rightness of their view. Apparently, she will tolerate discomfort in college and maybe learn something new, if not about them, then perhaps about herself. As I bring an end to my thoughts of mice and men, I bid the class a good homecoming. This weekend, our football team will challenge the fighting team from another Midwestern university. It will be a gladiator's duel of honor for the benefit of those who have come home for the weekend.

Football Saturday is a grand time. I get up early and complete necessary Saturday "honeydew" tasks: "Honey, do this. Honey, do that." I've lived in this small apartment for seven years and I will miss it. Janet and I have started to search suburbia for our first home. Our realtor has called us several times with leads of fixer-uppers that have just come on the market. He says now is a good time to buy what with interest rates probably going lower. But I'll miss this dump and the memories. I've grown comfortable here.

Janet's usual flat belly is bulging with signs of new life. I like it. In public places, I have the urge to point to my doings. After all, I sparked the growth all by myself and without the benefit of my canes. I did good. Poor Janet is buying ridiculous maternity clothing. She carries the baby well and looks great, but her body is expanding, her face is full, and she is beginning to waddle when she walks. Walking together, we must look quite the sight: waddle and plop-slide. Her regime of jogging has become a fast waddle-walk of half the distance.

Our marriage ceremony was small and intimate. It was held in the "park" at the Center and nature kept rain clouds away for most of it. There were about fifty present and only one seizure. The chairs were aligned perfectly by several of the Center's residents, and the Park was adorned with flowers and streamers. It was a standard marriage. Janet wanted us to read our own prepared vows, but I was able to talk her out of it. Anxiety really tightens my spastic speech muscles. I can utter a simple "I do" clearly and articulately even when I'm panicked. But I was afraid that if I anxiously read a long list of promises and adornments, there would be mutterings in the audience: "Did he say he'd perish her for the rest of his wife?" "He has an infernal dove for her?" "What is that about his kart and troll?" Bob Charles was my best man, and when I asked for the ring, he searched his tuxedo in earnest. Or perhaps, it was yet another example of British humor. I never can tell. Besides, we were both pretty hung over. I was surprised to find that Bob could throw a wicked bachelor's party. I was happy to discover my singing prowess had not diminished over the years. Elroy and Trevor will never forget the stripper, and I'll never forget the sight of Rusty strobing while she performed. We all, in concert with Rusty, strobed while she gracefully removed her clothes to the bump and grind music. I wish I had a picture of that.

Elroy took the marriage well. Janet and I were concerned about how he'd react, but he sat in the front row with a smile on that big round face and seemed to enjoy it. I was afraid he'd object, jump to his feet, and in desperation, drag her down the aisle and away. But he simply sat, watched and listened with that self-assured look on his face. Later, when the beautiful bride kissed him, he almost collapsed in euphoria. After the too-long kiss, I shook his hand but he never lost eye-contact with Janet. As usual, I was just a nuisance and easily ignored. I had an urge to pull his hand forward, swing it above his head causing him to flip and sprawl on his back. He's a cocky little bugger.

Game time is 11:00 a.m. Janet and I plop-slide and waddle to the stadium along with the swelling mass of students and boosters. It is a beautiful fall morning. Hundreds of oak and maple trees show their colors. Football Saturday is a carnival, and there is a magical crispness in the air. Today there are jugglers and minstrels performing for pocket change, tail-gate parties of drunken football fans, and the blimp floating above it all. You can hear the echo of the marching band. We give our tickets to the guard and manage to find our seats on the second story of the stadium. I see Bob has already arrived, and we greet each other. He offers us a sip of his brandy-spiked hot chocolate and remarks our team will again snatch defeat out of the jaws of victory. I suspect, because of the brandy, he got the statement backward, but then, with Bob, I really never know. Of course, alcoholic beverages are forbidden, but as tenured professors, we feel we have special privilege. Elroy and Janet share a sandwich as the coin is tossed. Our team elects to receive. We will accept the challenge.

Preponderance of Evidence

Although this story is based on an actual legal case, the specific corporations and facilities described herein are fictional, and resemblance of the characters and patients to any person, living or dead, is purely coincidental and unintentional. This story was originally published in *Exploring Communication Disorders: A 21ˢᵗ Century Introduction through Literature and Media (*Pearson Allyn & Bacon Publishers*)*.

Chapter 1

"Madam Forewoman, has the jury reached a verdict?"

A well-dressed woman in her early thirties stood in the jury box and faced the judge. Obviously nervous, but with a sense of resolve in her voice, she replied, "We have Your Honor. The jury finds for the plaintiff."

As sighs of relief saturated the oak and mahogany courtroom, the judge acknowledged the verdict by writing something on a small note pad. Then, for ten gratifying minutes, the forewoman continued to list the charges and verdicts against the defendants. The courtroom again resonated with sighs when the forewoman decreed that punitive damages should also be awarded. The final award would be in the millions.

Michael Blake and Margaret Hunter turned to each other at the plaintiff's table and hugged in relief. After the jury was dismissed, and the courtroom emptied, Mike and Margaret were greeted by Mason Sommerness, the senior partner and namesake of the firm. Mason lavished them with praise for a job well done and offered assurances of vacations, bonuses, and perks. "The mother of all cases," he called it.

The case lasted three years and just about financially gutted the small law firm. Expert-witness fees, travel costs, depositions, autopsy reviews, and expense after expense nearly depleted the firm's resources. Last month a bridge loan from a friendly bank had kept salaries forthcoming for the office staff. Fortunately, there would be no appeal, and within six weeks, Mr. Albert Anderson's estate and the law firm of Sommerness, Blake and Magnum would receive their just rewards. For Mike and Maggie, month after month of 12-hour days would be rewarded. Of course, for both the firm and the family, the settlement was bittersweet. No settlement would return the spark of life that was Albert Anderson. No settlement would ever return him to his loving children and adoring grandchildren. Nothing would ever erase the memory of his unnecessary, premature, and tragic death. The huge medical industry defended his death and as yet another "acceptable" casualty. After all, he was in his 70s. After all, he was sick. After all, he had undergone heart surgery. After all, people die. But to the people who mattered, the judge and jury, Albert Anderson's demise was the result of an arrogant, uncaring, negligent nursing home and a series of sloppy medical decisions. The nursing home and its larger, deep pocketed parent company, Southwest Healthcare Systems, would pay dearly for his death, and just maybe because of it, future lives would be saved. Albert Anderson's death would not have been in vain. As Mike told the jury in the summation, "After all, people deserve better."

Three years ago, Nina Miller, a woman in her late 40s, entered Michael Blake's office and said her father just died. She talked about his heart surgery, depression, and loss of weight. She told of the months she desperately tried to help him. She spoke of the love she had for her "daddy," and told of the nursing home that had promised to help him gain weight and recapture his rugged, athletic frame. The grief-ridden daughter also produced a picture of Albert Anderson proudly sitting atop a horse, with snow and pine-covered mountains in the distance, apparently taken two years before his death. She also showed Mike the nursing home brochure which boasted of its ability to help people like him. Then, Nina told him a woeful tale of misdiagnoses, broken lines of communication, improper care, indifferent doctors and nurses, and a nursing home that didn't give a damn. As she sobbed quietly, she told of an emergency room doctor, who upon seeing her emaciated father, threatened to call the police, to bring charges against her! When she told the ER doctor that she was bringing him from a local nursing home, Palo Verde Eldercare, he had uttered the word "criminal." Two days later, Anderson died a death of starvation, fever, and suffocation. He drowned in his own fluids, and his heart gave out.

At first, Mike had agreed just to look into the case. He knew this would be a big commitment and the financial risks to the firm would be substantial. At 53 years of age, Mike was comfortable. After years of struggling, his practice had blossomed into a small, but secure firm specializing in accident and disability law. He still worked long hours but enjoyed what he did. A new home had just been purchased and a grandchild was on the way. So, he decided, he would begin with a simple look-see. He would test the legal waters carefully before committing his firm's future.

His first stop was the emergency room and a quick discussion with the ER physician. The doctor remembered Mr. Anderson and confirmed the report by the daughter. A review of the medical records showed his weight to be 97 pounds; his height was five feet, eleven inches. The county pathologist also remembered Anderson's body and the "infiltrates" found in his weak lungs. Death was listed as congestive heart failure. The pathologist also remarked that something was medically awry. Something was not right in the death of Albert Anderson.

By the end of the month, Mike and his legal secretary and investigator Maggie, had completed their initial investigation. There were several tense meetings with the staff and other partners of the firm. On a Friday afternoon, at precisely 4:15, they met with Nina and agreed to take the case. On behalf of Albertson Anderson's estate, the small law firm of Sommerness, Blake and Magnum would sue two physicians, the administration and medical staff of Palo Verde Eldercare and its parent company Southwest Healthcare Systems. David would take on Goliath.

Chapter 2

Kendra Coons, Corrine Erickson, Seth Stubblefield, and two assistants, were the entire Speech-Language Pathology Service for the 230-bed hospital and the two adjacent nursing homes, one which had been purchased by the parent company Southwest Healthcare Systems. As recently as two years ago, their department was double that size, but corporate, insurance, and Medicare changes resulted in personnel cutbacks. To say they were overworked and understaffed gave new meaning to the word *understatement*. But, as Kendra said at the close of each weekly staff meeting, "Ours is not to question why."

Corrine and Seth, with the help of the two speech-language pathology assistants, did the majority of evaluations and therapy for the inpatients and outpatients at the hospital. Kendra, as chief of the service, had some clinical duties, but about fifty percent of her time was taken by important and not-so-important administrative responsibilities. With the acquisition of the adjacent nursing home, Palo Verde Eldercare, or PVE as the staff was now calling it, she had assumed some clinical transition duties. Prior to the acquisition, PVE relied on private contract suppliers of speech-language pathology services. Understandably, the private practice group was unhappy at losing the nursing home contract, but was cooperative and helpful during the recent transition period. Actually, Kendra was impressed at their professionalism and the way they put the patients' needs above all other concerns during this difficult and awkward period. Kendra hoped she, and her overworked staff, could continue to provide high-quality services for the 66 residents of the nursing home.

Kendra was approaching retirement age. Although the idea of unlimited days of golfing, traveling, and gardening was appealing, she knew she was not one who could idle away time. Time was too precious. Her professional life had been too full, too rich, and too rewarding. Kendra knew, for her at least, the so-called golden leisure years would be a fool's gold paradise, dull and boring without the professional stimulation to which she had grown accustomed. Her profession was too much a part of her life to simply walk away and not look back. It wasn't a matter of money, either. Several bull markets, a diversified 401K plan, and her disciplined monthly IRA investments had paid off. Kendra was a wealthy woman. She still had three years to ponder options and possibilities, and in the back of her mind, she added part-time private practice to them. Ah, to be her own boss.

Corrine and Seth made a great team. The two saw eye to eye on just about everything related to the practice of speech-language pathology in a medical setting. This was even more remarkable given their different educations. Corrine took the standard route to the profession. Early in her undergraduate career, she declared it as a major and she was accepted into graduate school on the first try. With an undergraduate GPA of 3.93 and an excellent GRE score, Corrine could have had her pick of graduate schools. However, a bearded young man, a biology major, and passionate love interest at the time, made it an easy decision to obtain both degrees from the same university. Maslow's hierarchy held true for 22-year-old Corrine. Love needs outranked all but safety and breathing on the road to self-actualization. Besides, it was an old and obsolete dictum that the graduate degree should be obtained elsewhere from the undergraduate one. With faculty turnovers, the revolution in information technology, and the fact that the American Speech-Language-Hearing Association reviews and accredits graduate programs, one can get a fine education without jumping from one university to another. And, most important, Corrine had her whole future to consider, and the engagement ring had been a major part of the equation. Sadly, whether it was the result of the stresses of graduate school or a difference of opinion about the important things in life– children, religion, and where to set down roots— their future died a quick but painful death. To Corrine, the final year of graduate school was saturated with the grief of their lost future together. And in many ways, a future is the hardest to lose. The passage of time, her first professional job, and a move to the Southwest had healed much of the pain, as had a tall, soft-spoken computer analyst who worked in the hospital's business office. Time helped Corrine realize there are many wonderful roads beside the one not taken.

Seth's path to the profession was nonstandard to say the least. It seemed he just couldn't find a major that suited him. At the end of his junior year, he had finally majored in "general studies" as a desperate attempt to get a degree in something, anything. His advisor told him it was a fine, liberal-studies type of education sought by many employers. Today, employers simply want to train their own employees. The seasoned advisor also confided that many juniors and seniors have yet to commit to a lifelong career. And perhaps, even the idea of committing to one discipline for an entire lifetime was as dated as the required blue suits and corporate allegiance to IBM, and other paternalistic megacorporations, in days gone by. After all, learning had become a lifelong pursuit opening up many new employment possibilities. When Seth's father suffered the massive stroke and lost his speech, his lifelong learning path took yet another detour. In the eight months before his father's death, Seth had a crash course on the nightmare that was aphasia. The massive stroke took his father's language, but it also sparked an interest in this mysterious disorder. After taking "leveling" courses, Seth was admitted to a graduate program in communication disorders. Three years later, he found himself working with hundreds of patients with aphasia, all trying to navigate through a wordless world. Seth finally found his calling.

Chapter 3

Helen Cutler is a delightful woman and Seth looked forward to the 50 minutes, a clinical hour, spent with her. A clinical hour is 50 minutes of direct patient contact, and ten minutes to chart the SOAPs. Subjective, objective, assessment, and progress was the structure the progress notes were to take when written in the chart, and everyone knew the job wasn't done until the paperwork was completed. However, over the years, the clinicians had stopped the formality of carefully identifying the patient's status and progress in SOAP form, and now three or four lines on the yellow "Speech Pathology" notes sufficed. SOAPS had evolved to a simple short paragraph, to no one in particular, showing what goals and objectives are being sought and how well the patient is responding. And Helen is improving like gang-busters.

Helen always dressed for therapy, much like she dressed for dinner. The 86-year-old suffered a stroke which caused the right side of her face to sag. Her tongue movements were slow and sluggish, and, at first, she sounded like she was talking with a mouthful of peanut butter. However, Helen was more concerned with the drooling. Her self-esteem could handle the slurred, distorted speech, but the saliva that dripped from her mouth was most disconcerting to her. It was too unladylike, and Helen is the consummate lady. Her hair is always sculpted impeccably, and her face adorned with just the right amount of makeup. There is just the slightest wisp of perfume as she gracefully takes her seat at the therapy table. Fortunately, therapy and nature's healing ways stopped the drooling and cleared her mouth of the peanut butter speech. Helen was to be discharged soon, and both she and Seth were pleased with themselves. The therapy for Helen was a standard fare of muscle-strengthening exercises and sound precision drills. Both Helen and Seth found interesting ways to do the drills and exercises, to keep them from being boring, childlike tasks. Seth felt the vibration of his cell phone and the numbers 111 indicated he had a visitor.

The woman introduced herself as an investigator with the law firms of Sommerness, Blake and Magnum and said she had a few questions for him. With those words, Seth's mental alarm went off. Up went his guard. She might as well have said she represented the Devil and was his senior Angel of Death. Seth wondered if he was being sued, and gratefully recalled that the hospital paid his, and the other clinicians, medical malpractice insurance. It was one of the perks negotiated before the layoffs. Two million dollars protected him, his sparse savings account, and future earnings, from the legal eagles, or vultures, depending on which side of the law you are on. Legal birds of prey and scavengers always seemed to circle a hospital. The attractive, well-dressed woman, Margaret Hunter, was professional, polite, and to the point. Did he remember a patient by the name of Albert Anderson? Was there ever a staffing regarding this patient? Did he remember a referral for a swallowing evaluation? Did he conduct one? Was a video swallow study conducted on the patient? Did he keep medical records in the department in addition to the ones in the patient's chart? Seth drew a blank. He told Ms. Hunter he would need time to consult his records. As he walked to his next patient, he thought, "Who the heck was Albert Anderson?"

"Is there anything worse than a brain tumor?" Corrine thought as she began the initial evaluation on the 37-year-old woman sitting in the chair. Her head was shaven, but new growth was just beginning to cover her scalp, which Corrine thought was remarkably smooth, and even attractive in an unusual sort of way. Would it be out of place to remark that even without hair, the patient was still a pretty woman? It seemed the baldness accentuated her dark brown eyes and full lips. She decided not to remark about the patient's appearance. Over the years, she learned that often the best thing said was nothing. As Corrine laid the test stimuli on the table in front of the patient, her mind focused on her own headache. "Great," she thought. "Now, I've got a brain tumor eating away at my gray matter." Of course, Corrine knew this was a psychological downside to the job. When you are around sickness and disease eight hours a day, five days a week, year after year, you don't have headaches, you have brain tumors. You don't mishandle eating utensils; you have early-onset symptoms of multiple sclerosis. The saliva on the pillow after an afternoon nap is an early indication of Lou Gehrig's disease. A little dizziness after standing up too fast is an impending stroke. Forgot your keys? Well, welcome to the world of Alzheimer's disease, where you meet new people every day.

Corrine went slowly with the patient. The evaluation would not be completed today, nor did it need to be. The patient tried her best to focus, but she was slow and often completely unresponsive. Even after completing the tests of her receptive language abilities, Corrine wasn't certain how much the patient understood what had been spoken. This was not the first patient she had evaluated with a brain tumor, and Corrine knew she would likely improve, often rapidly, after the surgery. Sadly, she also knew brain surgery often only bought time for the patient, a few more months and perhaps a couple of years. Of course, there was always room for optimism with the new generation of drugs showing so much promise in cutting blood supply to tumors and even attacking their evil genetic core. Corrine's role in the cancer battle was all about the patient's quality of life. Others would try to destroy the army of out-of-control brain cells. Her job was to help the patient regain as much communication as possible. Her job was to help this woman navigate the frightening changes in her speech and language abilities. Her job was to help restore speech and language and all the connections with loved ones that only communication can maintain. Her job was to make those additional years provided by the physicians and nurses as meaningful and rich as possible. No small task.

After completing the partial evaluation, she stopped at the cafeteria for a quick sandwich. It was 11:45 and Corrine was hungry; her stomach had announced it to all who rode with her in the elevator. After paying for the pastrami on rye and the diet drink, and automatically getting the generous employee discount, she took her usual table in the corner of the dining room, partially hidden by a huge support pillar. She liked to eat alone and cherished the time to read the latest mystery novel about a Navajo police detective named "Chee." But halfway through her solitary lunch, a woman approached her, apologized for the interruption, and began to ask her questions about a patient, Albert Anderson, of whom she had absolutely no recollection.

Chapter 4

At first glance, Palo Verde Eldercare looked like any other averaged-sized nursing home. Margaret Hunter had only been inside two other nursing homes in her life, and this one didn't seem much different from them. Not much different except for the odor, that is. It was a mixture of food, sweat, sickness, and old age. The place smelled dirty. The halls were lined with old people. Some patients shuffled slowly from one place to another, while others just sat in wheelchairs staring at her and into space. As she approached the first-floor nursing station, she noticed eight or ten people sitting in a communal television space, not really watching the old television set mounted high above their heads. The sound emanating from the television was too loud for normal ears, but probably too soft for them to hear. A perky talk-show host interviewed someone who felt deeply victimized by this, that, or the other fashionable thing. Tears flowed from the guest and an extreme close-up caught all of her talk show pain. The studio audience clearly commiserated with the poor, hapless victim, but for the residents at Palo Verde Eldercare watching the show, her plight— broadcast to millions of people and sponsored by a new and improved toothpaste— seemed trite. Maggie wondered if Albert Anderson sat in that same room, watching talk shows, wasting away, and silently passing time, until his days ended.

The Director of Nursing was defensive. Most people are defensive when talking to a lawyer or an investigator, especially when they are on the other end of the lawsuit. But this nurse was more defensive than most. She remembered Mr. Anderson and knew of his death. She also knew of the suit and had met twice with the administrator of the facility. She also met with the lawyers who would defend them, their action, and inaction. She provided little information about his medical condition, standard of nursing care for him, diagnostic procedures, or therapies. In effect, she told Maggie the only information she would receive about the case, at least from her, would be during a deposition or trial, under oath, and with her lawyers present. That was fine. After all, that is the way the system worked.

On the way out of the Palo Verde Eldercare, a nurse's aide approached Maggie and asked to have a few words with her. Lori, a woman in her early forties, a bit overweight but strong and muscular, wanted to talk about Mr. Anderson. After looking around for spies, they slipped into a vacant room. Maggie took notes while Lori spoke of Mr. Anderson's care, or lack of it, the indifference and incompetence in his treatments, and the thinly veiled frustration and anger many of the staff felt for him due to lack of improvement. She confessed she had grown to like Mr. Anderson. She also told of the "soup incident."

Chapter 5

After Albert Anderson's heart surgery, he began to lose weight and was depressed. These are not uncommon reactions after major bypass surgery. But Albert continued to waste away. After his surgery, his anxious daughter, Nina, brought him home and tried to nurse him back to health. She regularly consulted with his doctor and did everything she thought was right. She fed him slowly and carefully eight to ten times a day. She created a warm, bright bedroom and was vigilant about his medications. She loved, nurtured, prodded, and tried to coax him back to health. She happily returned the love he had so unconditionally given to her, but it was to no avail. He just barely held his own weight. Then, one day she saw an advertisement in a newspaper. A nursing home, not far from her house, professed the staff, skill, compassion, and expertise in helping patients just like her father. Three days later he was admitted to Palo Verde Eldercare. Nina finally sought help from medical specialists. She breathed a breath of relief. Unfortunately, that breath of relief quickly turned to a gasp of exasperation.

At first, Albert Anderson's medical care appeared competent. He was placed in a private room, and medical professionals from all walks of life evaluated, interviewed, and planned for his care. The paperwork was completed in great detail, especially those dealing with the out-of-pocket expenses she, with the help of a second mortgage on her home, would have to endure. However, within a week or so, Nina started to notice signs all was not as it appeared. Meal trays were just left with her father, sometimes out of his reach, and picked up later with nary a bite taken. He continued to lose weight. His depression deepened, and his antidepressants were given at irregular times, if at all. Frequently, an entire day would pass without Albert Anderson ever leaving his bed, except for the occasional trip to the bathroom, which required help from the scant number of busy, overworked nurse's aides. And more than once, to Nina's disgust, he spent hours laying in his own waste; the call light had repeatedly been turned off at the nurses' station. And then there was the incident with the soup.

It was no secret that Albert Anderson was allergic to milk products. Nina had told everyone about his serious allergy, from the attending physician to the nurse's aide who brought him his tray. It was listed in every section of his chart. She had even printed a sign and placed it on the wall of his room. Milk products had always caused her father to have a violent reaction, often requiring an immediate, panicky drive to an emergency room. So, when Nina had unexpectedly visited him at lunch time and found the bowl of New England clam chowder, loaded with whole milk and carelessly placed on his tray, she became furious. She immediately took the bowl of soup to the nurses' station. As she walked toward the three nurses and ward clerk, she got the usual unmistakable looks from them: "Here comes that pest with yet another complaint." When she showed the bowl of soup to one of the nurses and got the usual brush off, Nina simply threw the contents of the bowl on the counter. Five weeks later, a judge threw out the complaint from the two nurses who alleged of being scalded by the lukewarm soup. The judge boldly stated that the action of Nina Miller, although inappropriate, was understandable and possibly justified.

Nina, a hands-on kinda gal, was not reticent about continuing to complain to the powers-that-be about his lack of care. Oh, the nurse's aides listened to her and promised to do better. The nurses also said they would be more careful. The doctors assured her all was well. Even the hospital administrator reminded her that they, and not she, were the professionals and knew best. But nothing changed, and Albert Anderson slowly began to die.

Several times Nina had called The Doctor. Each time, it was a hurried, impatient, one-sided conversation. The Doctor was a busy man, and she understood that. He was also one of the finest heart surgeons in the Southwest, a fact she would never deny. After all, his skilled hands had repaired her father's heart. But he just seemed too busy to talk to her about pressing post-surgery concerns. Several times, she asked The Doctor if something might be wrong with Albert's ability to swallow, and several times, he said he would look into it. She got the same indifference from him as she did from the staff at Palo Verde Eldercare. As she told The Doctor, sometimes, when her father would eat, he'd panic and push the food away. But there were no signs of choking. He'd rarely coughed or gagged. After a meal, if you listened carefully, you could hear a gurgle deep in his chest. And he always seemed to have a low-grade fever.

So, to the medical specialists, if Albert Anderson didn't cough, choke, or gag, he obviously didn't have a swallowing problem. His refusal to eat, the occasional panic attacks during mealtimes, and loss of weight were common problems associated with post-surgery depression. Sometimes, Nina got the distinct impression that had she gone to college like everyone else in the medical world, she would have known this simple truth. After a while, she stopped wondering, aloud that is, whether her father had a swallowing problem.

Chapter 6

Had the results not been so tragic, the botched orders could have been called a comedy of errors. On a chilly day in November, The Doctor had his nurse call in the orders, and the busy charge nurse at Palo Verde Eldercare dutifully noted them on the chart. No one will ever know for certain whether The Doctor's nurse misunderstood his words or whether the charge nurse at Palo Verde Eldercare made the mistake, but an upper GI was ordered rather than a video swallow study. No one will ever know for certain whether The Doctor referred Mr. Anderson to the speech pathology service for an informal speech and language evaluation or whether he wanted a comprehensive dysphagia assessment. All that was written in the chart was "speech referral." No one will ever know for certain why Mr. Anderson didn't get a complete, comprehensive swallowing assessment. However, one thing was known for certain by the plaintiff's expert witnesses who testified three years later. Mr. Anderson was silently aspirating deadly food particles into his lungs for weeks, perhaps months, before his death. And to one expert witness, a physician with a medical degree from a fairly decent school, Harvard University, those particles led to the congestive heart failure that killed Mr. Albert Anderson.

That Mr. Anderson didn't choke, gag, or cough during meal times did not rule out a swallowing problem. Silent aspiration occurs when a patient appears to swallow normally, but food particles or liquids are breathed into the lungs. Usually, in silent aspiration, the patient swallows, but some of the food particles or liquids remain in the throat, either at the base of the tongue or around the vocal cords. Then, when the patient breathes after the swallow, the particles are sucked into the lungs. This problem is compounded if the patient doesn't have a productive cough. Often, weak and feeble patients can't build up the air pressure to blow the aspirated food particles from their lungs or the passages leading to them. It is called silent aspiration precisely because the patient doesn't cough, choke, or gag. It is a serious medical condition, which often leads to pneumonia, and it can be deadly.

There are several steps to a comprehensive swallowing evaluation. Usually, it is preceded by a bedside assessment. Here, the speech-language pathologist assesses the patient's oral-motor abilities and sensation. But there is only so much information that can be obtained at a patient's bedside. If the clinician suspects the patient may be silently aspirating, he or she recommends the barium swallow study and actually goes to the Radiology Department to participate in the procedure. After donning lead aprons to protect from the radiation, the clinician watches as the patient (actually his or her blurry skeleton) swallows a white liquid and other foods soaked in the stuff. During the procedure, the clinician can see whether the patient aspirates during any aspect of the swallow. Although there are false-positive and false-negative results to any medical tests, the majority of the expert witnesses opined that Albert Anderson would have survived his dysphagia had this procedure been followed.

Chapter 7

The depositions were taken in the Gold Conference Room of the hospital. Corrine, Seth, and Kendra were scheduled, in that order, to take a solemn oath to God that everything said was the truth and the whole truth. They agreed to provide all they knew about Albert Anderson. The depositions for each clinician lasted about an hour, but they were very long hours. The defendant's attorneys were present and conferred, objected, and moved to "strike" regularly during Mike's examination. Mike was always pleasant, but very businesslike, as he sought to get to the truth. A court reporter took down every word, every "ah," "um," and stutter in frightening detail. By noon, Corrine, Seth, and Kendra were deposed and deposed well. Other depositions were taken that day and even more were scheduled at different places and different times. Nurses, nutritionists, social workers, doctors, administrators, and family members all experienced the ordeal of the deposition.

During the trial, neither Corrine, Seth nor Kendra were required to testify, although their depositions were referred to several times. Lori, the nurse's aide, was examined and cross-examined for six grueling hours. Michael skillfully re-created the series of events that led to Mr. Anderson's death. Breakdown after breakdown in communication occurred between The Doctor and the other medical professionals. Mike proved, beyond a reasonable doubt, that the standard of care for Mr. Anderson was certainly inconsistent and inadequate. He created an accurate picture of Palo Verde Eldercare as a shoddily run, negligent nursing home. Although most of the staff tried to provide quality care, the nursing home's motivation for profit often torpedoed their efforts. Mike also showed how a patient like Mr. Anderson, who fails to improve as expected, can sometimes create a culture of resentment and negativity among the medical staff. This is especially true when there is stress and conflict with a family member. He told of the soup incident. Mike clearly portrayed The Doctor as a skillful surgeon who dedicated his life to help the hurt and sick, but Mike also showed that The Doctor was not careful enough, nor did he keep up on important post-surgical medical treatments and therapies. And Mike provided a preponderance of evidence to the jury of seven women and five men, with two alternates, that the speech pathology staff never did get the referral on Mr. Anderson. They were never able to do the testing and therapies that "probably" would have saved his life. In the legal world, the distinction between "possible" and "probable" is an important one.

The orange, desert sun set over the top of the modest homes. Children laughed and played. Finally, it was beginning to cool down, and the thermometer only read 99 degrees. Of course, it is a dry heat, as if that's a comfort to desert dwellers. Nina Miller had just finished pouring herself another glass of sun tea, which had been brewing all day on the porch, when she saw a red, Pontiac Grand Am pull into her driveway. Maggie Hunter, dressed in a comfortable sun dress, politely refused the large glass of iced tea and told of pressing after-work shopping that needed to be done. Then, Maggie pulled from her purse a very formal looking check and gave it to Nina. The check, written to his estate, and the first of three to be delivered by Maggie, had five zeros behind a single digit. Both women began to cry. Later, as the red car drove off, and the tears dried on her face, Nina sadly returned to the kitchen of her modest home. As she looked in the direction of the vacant bedroom where she had tried so desperately to nurse her loving daddy back to health, she knew how empty this victory really was. She would gladly tear up this check, or any check, even one with fifty zeros behind double digits, to hear the laughter and see the smile and to be hugged, just one more time, by her daddy.

A Day at JFK

This story was originally published in *Exploring Communication Disorders: A 21st Century Introduction through Literature and Media* (Pearson Allyn & Bacon Publishers).

Ah, school days, school daze. Twelve years of desks, lunchrooms, chalkboards, friends, crayons, recesses, rejections, loves, loves lost, bullies, nerds, holidays . . . each day a drama for teachers and students alike. There are hundreds of cast members, each with their own script, and as they say in theater, there are no small parts.

What follows is a story about some of the teachers, parents, and students whose lives intersect at John F. Kennedy Elementary School. Take a few minutes and read about the best of times and the worst of times for Alex, a child who stutters; a young boy and girl with delayed language; little lisping Blake; and Kevin, a child born with a cleft lip and palate. See what it is like to be young and different when it comes to communication. Meet children with articulation problems, and Wendy, a speech-language pathologist, whose job it is to help all of them. See how communication disorders affect these children, their parents, and classroom teachers every day at JFK and thousands of schools just like it.

Alex

You can hear a pin drop. Try as he does, Alex cannot look up from his brand new white running shoes. They are the kind with red lights that flash on the heels every time he steps down. His mother was not happy about their cost and had said something about having to get second a mortgage to pay for them. Alex had no idea what a mortgage was, but he suspected it might be where parents get money for kids' shoes. (Maybe a third mortgage will pay for the 21-speed mountain bicycle he saw in the window of the Broken Spokes Bicycle Shop.) As Alex stares at his shoes, he wishes they could somehow magically transport him from the front of this classroom to his tree house high atop the backyard oak tree. The silence is deafening. Finally, he hears some kids at the back of the class talk and laugh, and he knows it is about him when he hears the whispered words: "Porky Pig." His stomach tightens into a knot.

Mrs. Lawson also feels the tension and wonders how to handle the situation. She knows Alex is going through a stage in which he stumbles and struggles with his speech. Over the years, she has seen many of her pupils repeat and hesitate as they speak in front of her first grade classroom. But Alex is having more trouble than most, and she has never had a child just stop in the middle of a sentence and stare at the floor. "Thank you, Alex," Mrs. Lawson says more to the classroom than to him. "Children, it's only ten minutes until lunch break. Return crayons to your cubby and get in line for lunch." In an instant, the quiet of the classroom is transformed into the familiar sounds of first graders talking, milling, and laughing as they prepare for lunch. Some children reach for plastic lunch boxes with their names boldly printed in black marker, while others grasp stained brown bags. Meal tickets are pulled from the tiny pockets of children whose parents prefer they eat a hot lunch.

As Alex walks to his cubby, his shoes flashing red lights with every step, Mrs. Lawson asks him to come to her desk. She can see the embarrassment on his little face and wishes she had never asked him to present his "show and tell" to the rest of the class. But what was she supposed to do? All of the other children stood in front of the class and proudly told of pets, toy cars and trucks, leaves, and unusual mechanical objects. Alex brought the "bug in a jar" to class and to have never given him the opportunity to share the adventure of capturing it would have drawn even more attention to his speech problem. She tells Alex how well he'd done and pretends to be fascinated by the black-and-yellow bug.

Lunchtime at John F. Kennedy Elementary School starts at 11:15 a.m. and ends at 1:00 p.m. when the "commons" area is finally vacated. Row after row of chattering children walk through the cafeteria as food servers plop, stack, and pour federally subsidized meals to them. Kindergartners can barely reach the top of the serving counters and many sixth graders have already outgrown the tables. There is no shortage of energy as hordes of children fall upon the common. Lunch time at John F. Kennedy School is a treat for all of the senses. Today, the smell of loose meat, tomato sauce, milk, and bread saturate the area, as do the sights and sounds of youngsters learning and exploring everything new.

Steven stakes out a place at the lunch table for him and his friend, Alex. His jacket, lunch box, and 49ers cap are placed on it to clearly deter other children from sitting there. Alex is always late getting to the table and as usual, it is Steven's job to claim it. Steven and Alex's friend, Stacy, looks in his direction as she and her usual group of friends walk to the end of the long lunchroom. Although they are neighbors and often play together on weekends, Stacy has little to do with them during the week. She prefers her girlfriends, and that is just fine with Steven and Alex. To the boys, groups of girls are as foreign and strange as aliens from another planet. Stacy is fun to play with alone, but when she is with her friends, it is just too complicated. Besides, Steven and Alex have a serious problem to deal with this high noon. There is a stranger in town, and he apparently wants to befriend them. His name is Kevin. This is the third day in a row he sat next to them at lunch. It is time to see what this stranger is all about.

Kevin

Brent and Maggie Byrne moved from California last June. Both quit high-paying jobs and pulled their children out of excellent schools to leave the Golden State. Like thousands before them, they had grown tired of the California stress. Certainly, California is a wonderful state, an economic powerhouse. The state is blessed with warm temperatures, theme parks, the Pacific Ocean, and huge, sprawling centers of culture. There was never a weekend when the Brynes wanted for something to do. But California had been too much. There are riots, recessions, mud slides, earthquakes, floods, crime, and worst of all, mile after mile of gridlocked freeways. It was just one thing after another, and they finally had enough. After searching maps, travel brochures, and taking several "scouting" trips, they finally settled on this small town and the simple life it promised. One of the first lessons they learned was that the simple life was often accompanied by culture shock. It was amazing how many services they had taken for granted which were simply not available in small towns. One of the biggest concerns was the special needs of their seven-year-old son, Kevin. He was born with a cleft lip and palate.

It was seven years ago that Maggie breathed a sigh of relief as she literally counted fingers and toes. It wasn't until she looked carefully into Kevin's face that she saw the gaping hole; it extended from his lips to the back of his throat. It was certainly a shock, but she already knew nothing would ever detract from the love she felt for this little, helpless baby. She glanced at Brent and no words were spoken . . . no words needed to be spoken. As if with mental telepathy, they both communicated their resolve to love this child not only in spite of, but in many ways because of his facial anomaly. And Kevin had proven to be a little trooper. Although he suffered surgery after surgery to bring his lip and hard and soft palates together, he did little crying and even less complaining, especially considering what he went through. The surgeries and the weeks of healing were painful for Kevin physically and for Maggie emotionally excruciating. The earaches Kevin had every time he got a head cold had almost been as painful as the surgeries, but the tubes put in his ears by the otologist had helped. Maggie quickly learned that frequent earaches are also a part of cleft lip and palate.

The cleft palate team at the Children's Hospital was the most professional group of people Maggie and Brent had ever known. Surgeons, dental specialists, audiologists, pediatricians, speech-language pathologists, social workers, and psychologists met regularly with the family to review and plot the course of Kevin's habilitation. It seemed every aspect of Kevin's life had been considered and every problem related to the birth defect anticipated. The plastic surgeons were the ones who brought the most visible changes. It was wonderful how "normal" Kevin's face and mouth had become. With the help of dental braces, his teeth were also moving normally into place. Now he looked like many of the children at this small school, with shiny metal braces and rubber bands bulging from their mouths.

Although the surgeries to repair Kevin's appearance were in the category of a miracle, the ones to repair the soft palate and the way it moved to the back of the throat on certain sounds had not been as successful. Kevin still spoke with too much nasality, and they could often hear a "sssss" coming from his nose. It was left to the speech-language pathologists to help Kevin's speech sound normal. The gains in this aspect of his cleft lip and palate habilitation were slow, but they were happening nonetheless, at least while they lived in California. It was still an unknown what this small town would bring. Maggie and Brent were surprised to find there was no cleft palate team and there had never been one. It appeared Kevin was the only child in this rural community with this type of problem. As their new pediatrician noted: "We never had a need to create a team." She convinced them that although they had a different way of doing things, Kevin would continue to get very good care.

Steven and Alex look over at Kevin. Without a second thought, Steven asks: "May I have one?" He points to Kevin's "Eatables."

As Steven mooches the food, Alex thinks, "The new kid's got style." He looks over at the latest rage in first-grade lunches. It is a box with all the fixin's. All a kid has to do is to put the stuff together and, bingo, there is a sandwich, pizza, or Mexican meal. Alex brought "Eatables" to school a couple of times earlier in the year, but his mother said they were too expensive and had once again commented about going to the mortgage store for money. In a generous gesture to Steven's question, Kevin pushes the box in his direction and tells him to help himself. Steven, never one to turn down another kid's meal, finishes it in seconds. After a few first-grade pleasantries are shared, the three of them run down the stairs to the playground for a quick ritual of "prowl the yard." The friendships made that day would last for years. After the threesome broke to attend the afternoon classes, Steven remarks that the new kid is nice but seems to have a funny accent. Maybe he is from the Deep South. Alex figures he had also been in a bike accident, what with that scar on his lip. That is all they ever said about Kevin's cleft lip and palate.

Michelle

Michelle is a sweet child. She opens her heart to everyone, but especially loves that cat. The sight of her carrying that big, black-and-white neutered tomcat from room to room brings a smile to everyone who sees it. Michelle had always been smaller than the rest of her friends and how she manages to carry him from room to room without assistance is amazing. The fact that Michelle has cerebral palsy makes the feat even more remarkable. Michelle and that cat look quite the sight . . . this tiny girl carrying a huge cat, sometimes with his feet and tail dragging. You just can't hold back a smile when you see the look on that cat's face. It is one of benign feline tolerance. He obviously doesn't want to be girl-handled, but somehow he accepts the violation as his "job" in the family. He runs from everyone else, but not from Michelle. She loves that cat: a warm doll with fur and a heartbeat.

Michelle's cerebral palsy is mild, and according to the doctors, it is the type that would primarily affect her walking and talking, or motor skills, and then only a little bit. Jim and Cathy went through the expected emotional roller-coaster ride when the news was given to them. But over the past eight years, they learned to accept her disability and the day-to-day inconveniences it brings. She can get around without a wheelchair or walker, feed herself, go to the bathroom, and brush her long, reddish brown hair without much help. It takes a little longer and seems to be more awkward, but she gets the jobs done. Her speech patterns are typical of this type of cerebral palsy; sounds and words are slooooly draaaawn out as she forces spastic muscles into speech positions. To strangers, her slow, drawn-out speech sounds abnormal, but to Jim, it is music to his ears. After three strapping boys, this delicate, loving child is the apple of his eye. Jim and Michelle have that special father-daughter relationship and the cerebral palsy only makes it more special.

The realization that Michelle was also delayed in her mental abilities didn't happen suddenly; it took years for Cathy's nagging suspicions to be confirmed. Michelle just didn't do little things that Cathy had seen the other children do, or they were done much later. From holding her head up when she was an infant to the extra eight months it took for her to say "Mommy," Michelle appeared slower than Cathy's other children. At first, she just assumed it was the cerebral palsy, a result of the spastic muscles' refusal to move as easily as normal ones. But there was more to it than just the physical. Michelle's language development seemed different from that of the other children.

The first indication Cathy could not ignore happened when she was picking up Michelle from day care. When Cathy watched Michelle and the other children chatter about the class hamster, "Bud," the delay became apparent. The other children were putting three and four words together and even making adult sentences, but Michelle would point to the brown and white rodent and say, "Bud run." But the biggest indication that all was not well with Michelle's thinking was her lack of understanding. She just couldn't follow complicated directions. Although the other children her age had begun to follow step-by-step instructions, Michelle still seemed to get hung up on the first one. None of the day-care teachers said anything about Michelle's mental development but a conference with her kindergarten teacher revealed Michelle might be "mentally challenged." When Cathy was young, it was called "retarded," but now the words were "challenged" or "special." But Cathy knew what the words meant. Her youngest child, and only daughter, was going to have a more difficult life. For Michelle, the road to an education at JFK would be uphill.

Mikey and Nicole

Wendy, the speech-language pathologist, originally majored in education at a small northwestern college. It wasn't until her junior year that she realized she loved children but not classrooms full of them. Teaching a classroom full of children was different from teaching a child or a small group of them. She liked the individual contact. She wanted to make a difference. To Wendy, the one-to-one interaction was what teaching was all about. It didn't take her long to realize teaching a classroom full of 25 or more students did not lend itself to this close pupil-teacher relationship. She stumbled upon the major of speech-language pathology and audiology when there was a guest lecture in one of her education courses. Although Wendy was never impulsive, she formally changed her major by the end of that week, and she never regretted it. It took her an extra year to get the undergraduate degree in communication sciences and disorders, and she discovered that getting accepted into a master's program was very competitive. She was finally accepted into a small college in the Midwest, and two years later, she had the coveted degree. She did well on the national test and completed her clinical fellowship last year. The supervisor of her clinical fellowship was one of her professors who had been happy to travel to her small school for the site visits. He said that getting out of the academic environment once in a while was pleasant, and he looked forward to his visits to the real world. At last, she was a fully certified speech-language pathologist; a card-carrying member of the American Speech-Language-Hearing Association, or ASHA, as everyone called it.

Wendy looks forward to the morning sessions and is unhappy that a meeting would cut into them today. She particularly likes the time spent with Michael. Little Mikey has a language delay. The testing Wendy did found that, although he is as bright as can be in most areas, his vocabulary is significantly reduced. He just does not understand as many words as other children his age, nor can he use language to express himself as well as other kindergartners. The psychological testing done by the school psychologist showed his only problem to be with expressive and receptive language. After meeting with his parents, Wendy traced the problem to environmental deprivation. Actually, in many ways Mikey was far from environmentally deprived; he has a rich home life, full of stimulation. It just lacks enough interaction and communication with adults and other children. Mikey lives on a farm, a two-hour bus ride to school, and he has a pony, a pet goat, a large red barn, and acres of rolling countryside to explore. Mikey is an only child, isolated from other children, and is not developing communication abilities well enough. It is certainly a mild language delay, but a language delay nonetheless. Wendy knows little Mikey will only spend a few months in the speech program.

Nicole is a different story. Also a second grader, Nicki has a serious articulation problem. Wendy knows they are going to have a long-term relationship. At first, Wendy couldn't understand anything the child was saying. It never ceases to amaze her how well parents can understand their children, even the ones with major intelligibility problems. The first time Wendy met the family, Nicki had a long discourse punctuated with smiles, frowns, and expansive hand gestures. Unfortunately, all Wendy could understand were a couple of words in the long string of unrecognizable sounds. After Nicki completed the monologue, her mother turned to Wendy and matter-of-factly summarized: "Nicki said her little sister broke her ankle in a sledding accident." How Nicki's mother was able to decipher meaning from that unintelligible string of sounds still stuck in Wendy's mind. Over the months, Nicole began to learn the rules by which sounds were placed into words. Her speech was now beginning to be intelligible, even to strangers.

The IEP Meeting

"He's so ADD." Wendy turns to see a sixth-grade girl give the diagnosis to other girls who eagerly agree with her. As Wendy hurriedly continues on her way to the IEP conference room, she thinks of Mr. Palcich's sixth-grade class and wonders if he is now teaching a theory of disabilities module to the ten-year-olds. Then it hits her that the words *attention deficit disorder* are now like the word *neurosis*. ADD has entered the general vocabulary to refer to someone disliked or who creates problems. Actually, there are two types of ADD. There are children with attention deficits who are hyperactive and those who are not. Clinically, the classification criteria are hard to meet, and specific scores on tests and clear behaviors must indicate a child has ADD. Nowadays, it seems every child with a lot of energy is diagnosed by his or her parents, teachers, or sixth-grade girls as ADD. Wendy suspected both Tom Sawyer and Huck Finn would have similar diagnoses.

Individualized education plan (IEP) meetings are usually scheduled for late afternoon. Occasionally, there are necessary exceptions, and this morning's meeting is one of them. IEPs are important aspects of special education, and the faculty makes every effort to attend them. They are designated times when the professionals get together with a child's parents and discuss issues, plot a child's course of special instruction, and reviews progress. The meetings are usually held in the conference room– that is unless the Director of Resource Programs, Ms. Hacking, forgets to schedule it, as she frequently does. Wendy painfully remembers last month's IEP meeting held in a vacant classroom and how uncomfortable she was; adults were never intended to sit in those small classroom chairs. That meeting seemed to drag on forever. And there was the memorable exchange between Mr. Palcich and Ms. Hacking.

Bob Palcich is a sixth-grade teacher and has been one forever. Apparently, he thinks the computer-generated sign "Files Must Be Signed Out" prominently displayed over the rows of filing cabinets does not apply to him. Not only had he not signed for a child's file, but he had also taken it home for review, another no-no right up there with treason.

Whenever there are spats, Wendy, along with most of the team, just sits quietly and watches the drama. To Wendy, these dramas are rich entertainment, unless she is forced to be a participant. Mr. Palcich and Ms. Hacking had a lively discussion about procedures, confidentiality, responsibilities, tenure, "mindless bureaucratic rules" and seniority. Wendy had given both entertainers credit for a fine show, and considers the conflict a tie. By the end of the meeting, both had cooled down, with egos intact. Wendy knows Mr. Palcich will continue to take the unsigned files home for review, and Ms. Hacking will continue to object. There will be another act.

Wendy sits at the end of the conference table, opposite Ms. Hacking. Ms. Hacking is the consummate professional, and takes her job very seriously. Rumor has it that before being promoted to administration, she was one of the best resource teachers ever. However, in true Peter Principle form, she was taken out of the classroom and is now an administrator with the jobs of scheduling, budgeting, signing student files, coordinating IEP meetings, and participating in the inevitable one-act plays with Mr. Palcich and others. Although she performs her duties well, it seems she has to work very hard at them. According to the academic grapevine, teaching children with special needs had come very naturally to Ms. Hacking, much more naturally than administration. Wendy thinks it sad that good teachers are sometimes promoted away from that which they do best: teaching.

Mr. Palcich walks into the conference room. His mussed hair and shirttail hanging from his belt suggests he has already had a challenging morning. He smiles at Wendy and sits next to her. From his old, brown leather brief case, he pulls a handful of papers to be graded. He obviously is going to use the time before the start of the meeting to his advantage.

Bob Nettell is the school psychologist. Actually, he is the only one for the entire school district. He spends a lot of time on the road, traveling from school to school. The word for a traveling educational professional is "itinerant," and in rural communities, many people find themselves on the road a lot. Even Wendy has to travel to a small elementary school 30 miles away. On Tuesdays and Thursdays she leaves early in the afternoon in the school district's small, white gas-efficient car. At first, she resisted the "traveling speech show," but recently, Wendy has looked forward to the 40-minute trip. It gives her precious time alone, an opportunity to listen to the only rock station in earshot, at maximum decibel levels, and to enjoy the sights of the crisp fall foliage. Dr. Nettell spends most of his days in a similar car and she wonders if he listens to the same radio station. When he isn't traveling from school to school, he is stooped over papers, intensely scoring IQ, aptitude, and achievement tests. He is also getting that "spare tire" that goes with a sedentary job. Wendy took courses in college with aspiring school psychologists. She is convinced they view the entire world and all the people in it, in terms of standard scores, stanines, means, age-equivalents, and percentiles. They have a very statistical way of looking at things.

Marsha Marlow and Edna Hoopes walk into the conference room together. Edna is the resource teacher and Marsha the idealistic, enthusiastic student-teacher, a role she plays well. They appear to have developed a close professional relationship. Although Marsha is also from the small college where Wendy received her master's degree, they had not known each other. Most of Wendy's courses were in the College of Health Sciences and Marsha is in the College of Education. Marsha is learning a lot from Edna and many of the children in the resource room are benefitting from the additional personal contact. Marsha had also brought new information and ideas to this little school, especially on current ways of treating reading problems and how to handle kids with ADD, perhaps even that unruly sixth-grade boy.

The schedule shows the first child up for review is neither in Mr. Palcich's class nor in Wendy's speech program. Ms. Hacking has to make accommodations for this child's busy parents, both of whom are here for the meeting. To make room for the participants, both Wendy and Mr. Palcich sit in the not-so-comfortable couch next to the wall. The parents are understandably anxious and listen intently to the reports from the professionals at the table. The child is a bright boy with above-average intelligence. In fact, according to Dr. Nettell, he scored two-standard deviations above the average on a recently administered IQ test. Both parents breathe a sigh of relief when they are told this means he resembles gifted children more than average ones on most of the IQ subtests. He appears to do very well in school except for writing. He can't seem to put his ideas on paper. He has dismal spelling and struggles with all but the easiest writing tasks. His parents are happy he met the guidelines for inclusion in the resource program. He will leave his home room for an hour per day to get the special services he desperately needs.

The second child on the list is Alex. Wendy, leaving Mr. Palcich on the lumpy couch, takes her place at the table and prepares her notes. Mrs. Lawson and Alex's mother, Jan, enter the room together and sit next to the resource teachers. Wendy is happy the schedule is being followed and that Alex's IEP is to happen on time.

Alex's Mom

Jan had been concerned about Alex's speech for the past year. She hated to admit it, but she needed professional help in dealing with his stuttering. She was always independent about child rearing, and learning to speak correctly was no exception. In fact, when Alex had trouble mastering his /r/ sound, she had simply given him examples of how to say it and corrected him occasionally. Except for the stuttering, he now talked like other children his age. However, during the final few weeks of summer vacation, he stuttered much worse. She tried to help by telling him to slow down and think before he talked, but this seemed to make matters worse. Lately, he has been sounding more and more like her brother-in-law, who has stuttered all of his life. She actually welcomed the sealed note from the school speech pathologist requesting a meeting. She readily gave permission for the stuttering evaluation and had completed the long medical and educational questionnaire. She also filled out a stuttering questionnaire asking detailed questions about how many sounds he typically repeated, how long the stuttering silences were, and whether or not he struggled to get the words out. She answered them as carefully as possible.

During the short drive to the school's special education annex, Jan had to admit she was nervous about the meeting. She had never been to an IEP meeting. She knew she would be meeting with Alex's teacher, a school psychologist, the resource teacher, and Wendy, the school speech pathologist. Over the telephone, Wendy gave her some information about what was to be discussed and how IEPs worked, but this was to be a new experience for her. She felt more than a little intimidated. As she pulled into the parking lot, she realized her feelings were similar to the ones she had when she was a little girl in school. It was like being called to the principal's office.

Jan is greeted by Mrs. Lawson. They met briefly when she brought Alex to his first day of school. Jan was happy to learn Alex was going to be in her classroom. Mrs. Lawson had the reputation of being a superb first-grade teacher, and Jan knew how important first experiences and getting off to a good start are. They sit next to each other at the conference table as introductions are made.

Jan scrutinizes the people at the table, as she is certain they are scrutinizing her. They all seem pleasant enough as they are joking and taking with one another. As introductions are made, Jan is brought into the world of IEPs. She is also introduced to Dr. Nettell and a special education teacher. There is also a student teacher present. They share handshakes and smiles.

Ms. Hacking, the one doing the introductions and apparently the leader of the group, begins by reviewing Alex's file. They quickly get down to business. For the next 20 minutes, histories are reviewed, tests explained, opinions offered, goals established and refined, and problems anticipated. Like a morning fog, Jan's fears lifts as it becomes clear these people are genuinely concerned about her only child. He is not just another pupil, one of many. Every attempt is made to bring Jan into the discussions. Her ideas, observations, opinions, and feelings are sought by everyone at the table. But a lot of information is given, too. It was like a breath of fresh air to hear from Wendy and what she knows about stuttering. The goal is to detour Alex from the road to becoming a stutterer, one taken years ago by his uncle. The IEP team's professionalism also relieves the anxiety she has been feeling. Jan understands the long and short-term objectives she signed that morning are no guarantee of success, but she feels good about the steps being taken. With what she has learned, it all seems like common sense. As she leaves the parking lot that day, she feels relieved Alex is in good hands.

"On the Road Again"

Sometimes the speech teacher, who travels twice a week to his school, calls Blake out of class and they take that long walk to the speech room; other times, she simply sits next to him and helps with his desk work. Blake prefers the help with his desk work. He found the speech teacher also knows a lot about third-grade math. She spends a lot of time on numbers beginning with "his" sound, but she is also very helpful in getting the answers, too. "Six," "seven," "seventeen," "seventy" and "subtraction" are words she requires him to think about and occasionally repeat, and he is learning to make the "steam" sound like she wanted. All he has to do is to remember to keep his tongue behind his teeth. On the days when they work on "his" sound in the speech room, there are cards and computer pictures containing the /s/ sound. Sometimes "his" sound is at the first of the word, and other times it is in the middle or at the end. When he said "his" sound correctly, he usually gets praise from her in the form of a broad smile and a very sincere "Good job, Blake," "Good talking," or "Very good." He enjoys making her so happy by saying the names of the pictures correctly. He is certain he makes her day by talking with his tongue in the right place. If that is all it takes to make her happy, he would continue to do it. She is easy to please.

On the way back from the small elementary school and with the radio blasting, Wendy thinks about Blake. She always sees him at the end of the day because it is such a treat for her to work with him and she savors the moment. He sits so intently, hanging on every word she speaks, and does everything a third grader is capable of doing to produce the "sssss" so many children lisp. His improved speech is gratifying for Wendy, and she particularly enjoys the walk with him back to the noisy classroom. They talk of things important to third graders and so often forgotten by adults. From baseball to tall Trudy who taunts and teases him, Wendy relishes her brief window into the life of a third grader.

As Wendy pulls her little white car into the parking lot of John F. Kennedy Elementary School, she prepares mentally for the next day. Hopefully, tomorrow, there will be no interruptions of the morning sessions and the time she spends with Michelle and Nicki. Michelle will learn new concepts and how to manage spastic speech muscles. Nicki will learn the more advanced rules by which sounds are combined into words. She will work with Mikey on his nonfarm vocabulary list and with Kevin on talking with his mouth opened wider, a way of reducing too much nasality. And there will be the first session with Alex and her new mission to remove self-consciousness and struggle from this first-grader's speech. These children, and all of the others carefully placed on her caseload, will benefit from her knowledge, concern, and skills. As Wendy turns the lights off in her office and walks down the long hallway through the common, smelling the lingering, familiar smell of tomato sauce, she remembers that guest lecture about communication disorders and the career decision she made so long ago. She knows she is making a difference in the young lives with whom she has been entrusted. As Wendy walks to her car, she bids "Good evening" to Mr. Palcich, realizing he probably has yet another child's file hidden deep in that old, beat-up, brown briefcase. Tomorrow will be another day at JFK.

Welcome to the Cyber Speech and Hearing Clinic

This story was originally published in *Exploring Communication Disorders: A 21st Century Introduction through Literature and Media (*Pearson Allyn & Bacon Publishers*)*.

It is the not-too-distant future. The computer revolution that started in the late twentieth century still raged and showed no sign of retreating. No other device had changed humankind more than the silicon chip. It affected virtually every aspect of human life. Some of the changes demanded by the computer chip were painful, but many were wonderful as well. Medicine, science, education, religion, entertainment, friendships, business, industry, and family structures were all transformed by this tiny electronic device. The professions of speech-language pathology and audiology were no exception.

Nick and Jennifer sat quietly at the dinner table with little Andrea, their firstborn pride and joy. Lately, dinnertime with the small family had become too quiet, too lacking in communication. After weeks of concern, Jennifer decided something was wrong; all was not right with Andrea's speech and language development. At first, it was just a nagging suspicion that Andrea didn't talk as well as her playmates. Lately, the signs were more than Jennifer could ignore. While other children were making adult sentences and eagerly playing verbal games with one another, Andrea was distant and aloof. In communication abilities, Andrea seemed delayed when compared to other children of her age.

Quiet saturated the dining room as Jennifer reported her concerns to Nick. He listened intently as she spoke in excruciating detail of baby talk lasting too long, inabilities to follow verbal directions, and constant difficulties keeping up with other children at recess. Jennifer told Nick of her fear that Andrea might be delayed, or God forbid, retarded in her development. She anxiously awaited Nick's feedback while Andrea sat in her booster chair, silently making colorful sculptures with her food.

"You're right. Her speech development seems slow," Nick admitted both to himself and his young wife. "I've seen her play with other children, and she just doesn't seem to talk as well as they do. Maybe we should have her evaluated."

Jennifer found relief in his statement. At least Andrea's slow speech development wasn't just in her mind, a figment of her imagination. After all, Andrea was her first and only child, and she didn't have a lot of experience in these matters.

"Then it's decided," resolved Jennifer. "We'll get her evaluated as soon as possible."

Nick nodded and silently wondered how much the deductible and co-payments would cost, but his real fear was for his daughter and her future.

The next morning, Jennifer went downstairs to the most frequently used part of their house, the Cybercenter. It was a small but comfortable room, with brightly colored walls, large draping plants, and a thick, gray carpet. The computer was amazingly small given its capabilities. The big semicircular monitor was the newest digital brand. It went from floor to ceiling and almost provided a 360-degree viewing area. Jennifer sat at the keyboard and voice-response station while Andrea played quietly with her favorite robotic toy.

Jennifer's words, "On computer," were automatically voice-printed and immediately brought the big screen to life. From a directory of programs, games, and websites, she used the mouse to select the Cyber Speech and Hearing Clinic icon. One click later, a pleasant male voice announced: "Welcome to the Cyber Speech and Hearing Clinic. How may we help you?"

Jennifer replied, "I'm concerned about my daughter's speech development. She is three years old and doesn't seem to talk like other children her age." The computer voice acknowledged her concern and stated that a form must be completed before the evaluation could be conducted.

A few seconds later, a colorful form appeared on the big screen, and the computer voice stated: "Please complete this form. You may use voice or keyboard responses."

Jennifer began answering the questions: Child's Name, Age, Date of Birth, Method of Payment, Developmental Milestones, and Relevant Medical History. Permission was given to access the Cyber Pediatric Center's records for Andrea's medical history, including the brain scans that were completed on all newborns. Ten minutes later, the form was completed, and she clicked "Submit."

From her fifth-floor office in the modern-looking steel building, Angela, a certified speech-language pathologist, sat at her computer station. The morning had been typical, at least thus far. There had been the usual delays with public transportation, but she managed to arrive at work on time. After her usual cup of coffee, she consulted her computerized secretary to see what the rest of the day would bring. There would be four new evaluations, which had been scheduled in advance. Today, she was responsible for walk-ins. Walk-ins was an old term used to describe evaluations done without an appointment. The term originated from days of yore where patients physically came to speech and hearing clinics for unannounced evaluations. Of course, nowadays, it was rare that a clinician physically saw a patient either for an evaluation or therapy. It wasn't necessary. The computer extended the clinician's eyes and ears and could reach around the world, in an instant, to evaluate and treat a patient.

Angela preferred to wear the virtual reality headset. It was better than watching the large computer screen because she could walk around her office or sit comfortably in the soft reclining chair. The only disadvantage to the head set is that it always mussed her hair. Technology had come so far, yet the problem of mussed— or "virtual hair," as the teenagers were calling it—persisted. After getting comfortable, Angela commanded the computer to begin the new evaluation. The intake form, on a child by the name of Andrea, flashed on her big screen. Highlighted were certain terms the computer deemed salient. As Angela reviewed the form, she began the process of knowing this child's speech and language development. Then, the computer announced, "Beginning synchronsis viewing."

Immediately, the screen zoomed in on Jennifer, a woman in her early 20s. In the lower left part of the screen, a data frame listed the results of the intake questions for easy reference. Angela introduced herself and paused while a recorded message immediately provided her qualifications, license information, areas of specialty, continuing education credits, and other relevant professional information. Angela first engaged in the usual "chewing gum conversation" with the parent, remarking about the weather and current events. She also told the woman her physical location. Cyber clinics could be in any part of the country, or the world for that matter.

As Jennifer spoke, the professional information provided by Angela was displayed in written form in the lower left part of her screen. For future reference, it was automatically saved under the category of "Medical: Professional Information" in Andrea's health and medical files. There was never a need to delete information because storage memory was unlimited what with the new generation of computer technology. A recent development went beyond the silicon chip and stored memory at the atomic level.

Angela listened intently as Jennifer discussed Andrea's development. Each statement spoken by Jennifer was automatically evaluated for its truthfulness and arousal quotient. Key words spoken by her were selected and presented in the ever-changing data frames. Words such as *delayed*, *slow in development*, *immature*, and *unusual* were spoken with a high emotional content and identified in shades of red. After the initial conversation with Jennifer, Angela was aware of the distress this young mother felt over her child's communication abilities. She made a mental note to include intensive parental counseling and education modules as a part of the treatment program.

Jennifer was impressed with Angela and the way the interview was being conducted. After Angela had logged off, the formal evaluation began. On the screen, an older man with a pleasant voice appeared. He was a computer generated composite face and voice found to be comforting and professional. He asked Jennifer detailed questions about Andrea's cognitive, linguistic, and social-communication development. At the end of the parental interview, the completed form, and its profile charts with accompanying norms were presented in a data frame and merged into the appropriate section of the diagnostic report, which was constantly under construction.

The hearing evaluation was completed in less than a minute. As Jennifer held Andrea in her lap with the brightly colored headset and earphones snugly in place, the function and status of the external, middle, inner, and central hearing processes were tested. Clicks, tones, and buzzing sounds were the only things heard by Andrea. On a data frame, the completed hearing evaluation report was created, including colorful graphic charts of her brain and cranial nerve VIII. Andrea's hearing was tracked and evaluated from external ear to temporal lobes and she passed with flying colors. Angela remembered that in the past, a hearing test of this complexity would have taken hours, involved sound proofed booths, and complicated testing protocols; even then, its accuracy was sometimes suspect.

The direct speech and language evaluation tests were automatically chosen by the computer and they were adapted to Andrea's interests. The interactive tests used colorful cartoon characters who playfully asked questions of Andrea. As the talking dogs, cats, and chipmunks had Andrea remember, repeat, name, discuss, describe, and point, the computer analyzed and categorized each response. Andrea's cognitive, linguistic, and social-communication abilities were assessed using the latest tests. Phonological processes were identified as was the speed of motor responses and visual scanning times. Her length of utterances and vocabulary was computed in every possible way and charted in bar, pie, and line graphs. Everything from Andrea's cognitive-linguistic functioning to her metalinguistic awareness was assessed by fun-loving cartoon characters.

In the past, these types of tests were conducted by professionally dressed people. Test stimuli were formally placed in front of the child, and each response carefully noted with pencil and paper. Young children like Andrea were frequently intimidated by the strangers, and sometimes it was a crapshoot whether the final results actually reflected the child's communication abilities. Some children even refused to talk and clung to their mother's leg, crying. Angela chuckled to herself when she thought of the countless frustrated graduate students who had been required to write a diagnostic report based on the responses from a crying, nonverbal child.

Andrea's articulation was acoustically analyzed, and each sound compared to norms for intelligibility and precision for her particular language. It took years of research, but each sound produced by humans had been carefully analyzed by powerful acoustic instruments. The international project finally listed each sound in the 10,000 languages and dialects of the world and provided their specific acoustic parameters. Now, each sound spoken by a person was instantly analyzed and compared to norms, and a deficiency value given. The scores were provided for individually produced sounds and for ongoing speech. There were even separate intelligibility scores given when the listeners were family members, friends, and people unfamiliar with the child. The newest technology analyzed the articulation of people suffering from brain damage and neurological diseases, and not only acoustically determined the precision and intelligibility of their motor speech, but also identified the site and nature of the central nervous system damage. Although phonetics courses were still taught in graduate school, clinicians rarely used their ears to make judgments about a patient's articulation. Nowadays, the computer was simply faster and more accurate.

Voice parameters were also automatically profiled by the computer. Andrea's pitch, loudness, emphasis, shimmer, jitter, and voice-onset times were assessed and analyzed in seconds. The computer even noted early signs of progressive neurological diseases such as ALS, MS, and Parkinsonism. Early symptoms of these disorders often showed up in minor voice irregularities, and only the computer could detect them. Fortunately, medicine had powerful treatments which were more successful if they were caught early.

The orofacial evaluation was the final assessment. As the talking chipmunk asked Andrea to open her mouth wide and put her face close to the screen, the embedded camera noted salient facts about her tongue, lips, teeth, and palatal vault. Everything from tongue tremor to speed of ongoing oral muscular movement was assessed. A three-dimensional picture of Andrea's oral structures was created and added to the ongoing report. It highlighted structures and functions found to be nonstandard.

While the evaluation was being conducted by the computer, Angela was monitoring the stuttering therapy being provided to Matt, a fourth grader. With sensors attached to his fingers and wearing the EEG and brain-imaging "hat," he was provided with gradually increasing difficult sounds, words, phrases, and situations through computer interactive activities. One minute Matt presented a speech to a cyberaudience, and the next, he was ordered a soyburger at the local MacDougal's. The computer evaluated the tension in his voice and— along with EEG, brain imagery, and galvanic skin responses— it provided visual and graphic feedback about speech muscle tension and general levels of speaking anxiety. The computer gently guided him into more stressful situations as he learned to maintain proper levels of fluency and remembered to use his tools of fluent speech, which were automatically provided on the screen when appropriate. As Angela completed the minor adjustments of the stuttering program, the computer announced the evaluation on Andrea was completed.

The evaluation shown on the screen was complete in every detail. As Angela read it, she made minor additions and corrections to the report. Each deficient area of Andrea's speech and language evaluation was noted and the appropriate short and long-term objectives listed. The objective and treatment plans were detailed and specific, and had been chosen from thousands stored in the treatment banks. The report, with the parent's permission, would be automatically sent to Andrea's pediatrician and preschool. The Parent Training and Language Facilitation Program was loaded, and Nick and Jennifer would be educated, trained, and coached in childhood language development. The program chosen by the computer was specifically adapted to Nick and Jennifer's ages, education levels, and interests.

A simple click of the computer loaded the appropriate therapy program for each objective and merged them into a comprehensive treatment protocol. Andrea's preferred television and cartoon characters would be used as cyberfacilitators, and her favorite "great adventures" computer game would provide the theme for all therapies. Andrea's language development would improve as she played, talked, and interacted with the colorful cartoon characters. Daily suggestions would be sent to her parents and preschool teacher for their assistance in meeting the goals. Periodic reassessments were automatically given to the youngster, and adjustments made to the individualized education plan. Angela would regularly review improvement with parents and teachers, and adjust the treatment programs when required.

Eight months later, Nick and Jennifer again sat at the dinner table, this time trying to converse over Andrea's chatter. The sweet sound of little Andrea's normal speech and language was music to their ears. They talked about the improvement she had made in her ability to communicate as she talked on and on about the great adventure she and the fun-loving chipmunk had taken through the oak grove in the Cyberpark.